The Use of Self
in Therapy

THE *JOURNAL OF PSYCHOTHERAPY & THE FAMILY* SERIES:

The Use of Self in Therapy

Michele Baldwin
Virginia Satir
Editors

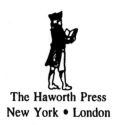

The Haworth Press
New York • London

The Use of Self in Therapy has also been published as *Journal of Psychotherapy & the Family,* Volume 3, Number 1, Spring 1987.

The Haworth Press, Inc. 10 Alice Street, Binghamton, NY 13904-1580
EUROSPAN/Haworth, 3 Henrietta Street, London WC2E 8LU England

Library of Congress Cataloging-in-Publication Data

The Use of self in therapy.

    Also published as: Journal of psychotherapy & the family, v. 3, no. 1, spring 1987.
    Includes bibliographics.
    1. Self. 2. Psychotherapy. I. Baldwin, Michele. II. Satir, Virginia. [DNLM: 1. Ego. 2. Psychotherapy—methods. W1 J0859C v.3 no.1 / WM 420 U84]
RC489.S43U87   1987   616.89'14   87-90
ISBN 0-86656-544-2
ISBN 0-86656-545-0 (pbk.)

The Use of Self in Therapy

Journal of Psychotherapy & the Family
Volume 3, Number 1

CONTENTS

Preface

Since 1900, much has been written on the nature of symptoms, approaches to therapy, therapeutic management, and the results of therapy. However, there is relatively little in the literature regarding the use of the self of the therapist in the therapeutic process.

We, the editors, hope that this issue will be a contribution toward that end. Through presenting the thinking and experience of persons who bring a historical, philosophical, clinical and research perspective to our subject, we hope to generate further interest on this vital factor. Rather than presenting a finished piece, we invite you to enter into an on-going dialogue with us, which we hope will enrich our understanding of the therapeutic process as well as the lives of therapists and clients.

The Editors

EDITORIAL NOTE

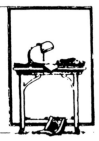

The *Journal of Psychotherapy & the Family* is pleased to present this special issue focusing on the therapist's use of self in psychotherapy practice. This collection is a fitting beginning for the third year of publication of the *Journal*.

The purpose of the *Journal* is to provide the practicing psychotherapist with a comprehensive array of well-written, accurate, authoritative, and relevant information vital to working with clients about interpersonal and family-related issues. Consistent with this mission, this issue of "The Use of Self in Therapy," edited by Michele Baldwin and Virginia Satir, is devoted to the practice of psychotherapy.

Here twelve scholars and practitioners address a fundamental issue in psychotherapy that is especially important in working with families: who am I in relation to my work and how do I and my fellow therapists use ourselves in the psychotherapeutic process? This is an important departure for the *Journal*. To date most of the attention has focused on the family system: its points of dysfunction and methods of intervention. Yet, our awareness of what we do as therapists, along theoretical and clinical lines, is subordinate to who and what we are to ourselves and to our clients.

The co-editors of this important collection, Michele Baldwin and Virginia Satir are both authors and family therapists. Dr. Baldwin is former Associate Clinical Professor of Psychiatry and Behavioral Sciences at the University of Nevada School of Medicine. She is currently a member of the faculty of the Center for Family Studies/Chicago Family Therapy Institute, Northwestern University School of Medicine. She has co-authored *Satir Step by Step* with Dr. Satir, led numerous workshops and has been a trainer in the Avanta Network. Dr. Satir is an internationally renowned educator and master therapist, a pioneer in the field of family therapy. She is Founder of the Avanta Network, Co-founder of the Mental Research Institute, former President of the Association for Humanistic

Psychology, and author of numerous books. Among these are *Conjoint Family Therapy, Peoplemaking, Self-Esteem, Helping Families Change, Making Contact, Changing With Families, Your Many Faces,* and her latest book, *Satir Step by Step,* which she co-authored with Dr. Baldwin.

As evidence of their world-wide esteem, they have been able to attract an outstanding group of scholars and therapists to write the most personal and practical collection of essays on the use of self ever assembled. Following an excellent and useful introduction to the collection by Dr. Baldwin, Dr. Satir contributes a touching and revealing essay on her views of the field of psychotherapy practice and the critical importance of the use of the deepest self of the therapist in empowering clients and opening up their healing potential.

Other major figures in psychotherapy practice match the important contributions of the editors. DeWitt C. Baldwin, Jr., Professor Emeritus of Psychiatry and Behavioral Sciences at the University of Nevada and currently the American Medical Association's Director of Education Research, contributes two papers, the first of which is a philosophical essay on the use of self. He first traces historically the concepts of self and concludes with an exposition of the parameters of self application by existential therapists. Carl Rogers, a true pioneer in clinical psychology and psychotherapy, then discusses his use of self in therapy and how it has changed over the years. David Keith, a Minneapolis psychiatrist and frequent collaborator with Carl Whitaker, writes of the supplanting of self in the process of psychotherapy training and discusses some methods for resurrecting the self, as he has done, over the years of clinical practice.

As somewhat of a counter-point to Keith, Bunny Duhl, Co-Director of the Boston Family Institute, who recently wrote the highly celebrated *From the Inside Out and Other Metaphors,* writes here of the importance of the use of self (both spatially and physically) and the development of self in psychotherapy training and practice. Another internationally renowned trainer, Harry J. Aponte, Director of the Family Therapy Training Program of Philadelphia, and Joan Winter, Director of the Family Institute of Virginia, also emphasize the importance of the *personal* aspects of treatment, as well as the technical aspects. They emphasize the importance of utilizing various contexts of a therapist's life—clinical, professional and familial.

Taking a different perspective, as he generally does, Alan Gurman, an internationally-known University of Wisconsin Professor of Psychiatry, Editor of the *Journal of Marital and Family Therapy* and of numerous important contributions, reviews available data which address the question of what constitutes an effective family therapist. Finding few answers, he makes suggestions for future programs of research which will, perhaps, answer these and other questions.

The editors conclude this important work on a humble note: rather than attempting to provide dramatically original and innovative viewpoints about the use of self in therapy, their goal is simple. They have attempted to provide a forum for leading therapists and scholars who, in different ways, plead for conscious recognition and awareness of the importance of the use of self in the therapeutic process and, thus, greater emphasis on the development and nurturance of this remarkable therapeutic tool.

Charles R. Figley, PhD
Editor

The Use of Self in Therapy: An Introduction

Michele Baldwin

At a time when many new forms of therapy and new techniques flourish it seems essential to more fully explore the role of the person of the therapist. This collection not only addresses how therapists use themselves, but also ways in which the "self" of the therapist can be used with more awareness and effectiveness. Several traditions influence the beliefs which therapists hold about the use of self. For example: the psychoanalytic tradition requires that the person of the therapist be as neutral as possible (Yalom, 1980). During the years following World War II, under the influence of humanistic psychology and of the human potential movement an opposite view emerged: the self of the therapist became an active ingredient in therapy, sometimes carried to the level of unrestrained self-expression and gratification. The impact of systems theory on family therapy has introduced yet another dimension. What then is the place of the self in therapy?

We are aware that this collection of papers will be controversial for several reasons. First, the subject matter: the entity of the self is a very personal matter. It also is elusive. We are not always aware when it operates, and when we become aware of its presence, its nature changes from being a subject to being an object of observation. In addition a "self" can never be known in its entirety, since others will never have complete knowledge of our inner experience, and we cannot observe some manifestations of ourselves that are readily perceived by others (Luft & Ingham, 1963, pp. 10-12). In spite of good reasons for some humility on the subject, we all have strong opinions about the "self" and how it should be used. Since these ideas are more connected with our emotions and belief systems than with our intellect, we are bound to react strongly to views which differ from our own.

Second, the format of this collection is unorthodox. In planning this monograph it seemed that the topic lent itself to a more personal style than is usual for an academic publication. Thus, several papers are written in the first person in an essay format.

Third, we were specifically instructed by the Editor-in-Chief, Charles Figley, that we were not to focus on family therapy alone, since the journal aims at a wider audience. At the same time we were aware that many readers may be looking for specific applications of the subject to family therapy. We would like to invite them to make and perhaps share these applications with us or in the literature.

Finally, although the papers in this collection represent a variety of viewpoints we have no papers opposing our thesis on the importance of the use of self. We accept that this reveals our bias and hope you will feel encouraged to share yours by communicating with us.

This collection intends to speak to issues affecting the practitioner, but it is not intended as a "how-to" manual on the use of self. Indeed, our concern is that "the use of self" could be construed as a new technique, as something that the therapist *does* in therapy. As stated by Yalom (1980): "When technique is made paramount, everything is lost because the very essence of the authentic relationship is that one does not manipulate but turns towards another with one's whole being (p. 410). This concern also offers a partial answer to readers who may question the validity of discussing together in the same collection of papers the use of self of the general psychotherapist and the family therapist. We are well aware that many family therapists who have broken away from the psychodynamic tradition may consider focusing on the experience of the individual as a therapeutic trap. They may feel that their concern about the use of self is of a different nature than that of other therapists. We wish to address this issue in several ways.

First, it seems important to acknowledge that any therapy, whether with individuals, families or groups, involves an interaction between at least two people. The focus is usually on the person of the client, who is supposed to have "the experience," with little attention paid to the leader of the interaction. Yet the person of the therapist always impacts the therapy. When the therapist denies this impact, he leaves out of his awareness a key element of the therapy. Also, as Yalom (1980, p. 404) points out it is easy to think that the client is responding to some specific technique, when the crucial variable may have to do with our humanness. We often underestimate the importance of the therapist-patient relationship and overestimate our cognitive contribution. Rogers goes further by stating: " . . . . Recently, I find that when I am closest to my inner, intuitive self . . . whatever I do seems to be full of healing . . . simply my *presence* is releasing and helpful" (Rogers, in press). In addition, if we focus on the characteristics of the dysfunctional family system, we usually find a lack of constructive feedback between family members regarding the impact of their behaviors on each other. When the therapist does not allow his own personhood to be present with a family, he operates under the same system as the family. When, however, the therapist uses his own reactions as a therapeutic tool, by sharing with the family how he is impacted by what is happening, and asking how his actions are impacting the family, he models a new way of operating which can effectively change the family system (oral communication by Virginia Satir, November 1985). Also as Shirley Luthman points out (1974), in the area of building relationships and intimacy, a therapist cannot take people where he has not been (p. 62).

Second, when it comes to the use of self, all differences do not carry the same weight. It is important to make a distinction between stylistic variables and core differences. Virginia Satir gave an illustration of these differences when we were reviewing Carl Rogers' contribution to this collection. She felt in agreement with everything he was saying—a core similarity—regarding their common belief in the sacredness of the individual, who posesses in himself the seeds for growth—and yet their personalities, techniques and ways of working are very different—stylistic differences.

The final point in this controversy comes from within the field of family therapy. As Richard Simon expresses it in the Family Networker (March-April 1986, p. 34): " . . . an increasing number of critics within the field have charged that our preoccupation with analyzing systems has led to a coldly mechanistic view of human relationships . . . . we have grown strangely distant from the struggle of individuals to find purposes in their lives . . . "

We do not deny that the family therapist may use himself in different ways than other therapists, and we are very specifically looking at ways in which family therapists use themselves. We only wish to point out that differences in personal characteristics may be more important to the effectiveness of therapy than differences in methods.

Our hope is to encourage reflection in the reader and to allow this topic to obtain the attention it deserves. We are not interested in creating controversy, but, rather, to stimulate the reader's thoughts. The question should not be whether the author is right or wrong, and whether or not you agree or disagree with him, but what is stimulated in you as you read. Are you raising questions about the way you work? Can you engage in a dialogue with the written material in a way that expands your horizons? We also hope that this collection will be useful to newcomers in the profession freeing them to be themselves, while alerting them to the dangers of the undisciplined use of the self.

This collection includes 10 papers written by psychotherapists with varying theoretical orientations who are concerned with the impact of the person of the therapist on therapeutic process and outcome. Two of these papers present a broad discussion of the topic, four papers describe the ways in which the authors use themselves in their practice, one describes a training program which integrates the training of the self of the therapist. Two papers are focused on research and the final contribution deals with the concept of the Wounded-Healer.

In the lead paper, "The Therapist Story," Virginia Satir takes an overview based on her experience and observations in forty years as clinician and teacher. This paper was initially intended as part of a joint introduction with Michele Baldwin. After it was written, however, we both thought that such a personal statement would stand better on its own. The paper starts by acknowledging the revolutionary contribution of Freud to mental health practice, then points out how, since the 1960s, the model of therapy has been expanded from the authoritarian doctor-patient relationship to include the patient as a partner. Next, Satir indicates the need to take into account the "self" of the therapist. Freud advocated that for the protection of the patient, the "self" of the analyst should remain neutral, and, to achieve this goal, mandated that he submit to a training analysis. Pointing out the damage that can be done by a therapist who is not aware of how he uses the self, Satir focuses on specific aspects of the therapist's behavior, such as how he uses his power, how he deals with his vulnerability, and how congruently he acts. Having thus alerted the reader to the dangers of the unaware self, especially in the misuse of power, she then states that the self of the therapist can and must be used to achieve positive therapeutic results. She views therapy as providing the context for empowering patients and opening up their healing potential, and states that this goal can only be obtained through the meeting of the deepest self of the therapist with the deepest self of the client. In concluding, she makes a plea that the "self" of the therapist be considered as an essential factor in the therapeutic process.

DeWitt C. Baldwin Jr., in "Some Philosophical and Psychological Contributions to the Use of Self in Therapy," gives an historical perspective to this collection. Although his paper may initially be a disappointment for persons strictly interested in a "how-to" approach, it will enable the practitioner to think through some key issues pertaining to the use of self in therapy. After a brief discussion of reasons why the concept of the use of self in therapy emerges at this time, the author looks retrospectively at the fascination concepts of self have held for writers and philosophers through the ages. He develops the viewpoint that is was not until Kierkegaard and the existential philosophers called attention to the world of subjective experience that the concept of the human being as both subject and object—as a self—emerged. Conceptualization of "self" excited the attention of philosophers such as Heidegger, clinicians such as Carl Rogers, sociologists such as George Herbert Mead, and theologians such as Tillich. This led to renewed interest in the "I/Thou" relationship, as posited by Buber, as well as in client-centered therapy as proposed by Rogers, both of whom place emphasis on mutual regard and respect between patient and therapist. After briefly reviewing the evolution of the concept of self in the works of Freud, Sullivan, Horney, Kohut and Arieti, Baldwin examines how psychiatry has been affected by changing views of neuroses since Freud and the emergence of existential philosophy. In this context he examines the works of Victor Frankl, R.D. Laing and Carl Rogers. He concludes by giving a description of the characteristics of the existential therapist for whom the use of self is an essential element in therapy, whether it be with individuals, groups or families.

The next four papers are by psychotherapists who discuss how they use themselves in their practices. First there is an "Interview with Carl Rogers on the Use of Self in Therapy," by Michele Baldwin. Rogers' seminal career has spanned over half a century of tremendous change in the field of psychotherapy. As editors, we felt that his perspective on his evolution as a therapist would be an important contribution to this collection. When approached, Rogers stated that he was unable to take on an additional writing commitment at this time. Because of his interest in the subject, however, he suggested the alternative of an interview. We were faced with the choice of foregoing his participation or accepting his contribution in the form he proposed, and decided to present this interview in the form of an essay. Rogers starts by pointing out his increased awareness of the use of self over time, and his own experience with use of self, including some of the risks involved. He then relates his views about related topics such as the therapist as a model, self-determination, transference, what constitutes appropriate goals for the therapist and the importance of maturity in the therapist. The middle section of the essay reviews the major turning points of Rogers' career and his evolution from a traditional therapist and academician, through person-centered therapy, to the present, where he is increasingly aware of the spiritual potential and dimension of the therapeutic relationship. This leads him to review the qualities of the authentic therapist, who, as a person, is both secure and aware of flaws which make him vulnerable. He then briefly comments on his views about the training of person-centered therapists, and concludes with a few words about what he believes his impact—or lack of it—has been in the fields of psychology, psychiatry, medicine, nursing and counselling.

The second paper in this group, "The Differing Self: Women as Psychotherapists" by Helen Collier, examines the use of self from a woman's perspective. Collier begins with a statement of her position regarding the myth of objectivity and reliance on scientifically replicable techniques in therapy. She views techniques as useful, but, in her view, the personal presence of the therapist is central to the therapeutic process. This personal presence, needs to be carefully monitored, however, because an unaware self can be dangerous for the therapeutic process. A high degree of consciousness is essential for the conduct of good psychotherapy. Collier then focuses on the main theme of the paper and looks at what being a woman means in that process. She bases her discussion on what Carol Gilligan calls the "different voice" of women. Gilligan claims that women perceive and constitute reality differently from men and that the two sexes are trained to experience and express things in a different way, masculinity being defined through separation and femininity through attachment. As a result, males tend to have difficulty with relating and females with individuation. Another difference lies in the way males and females conceive of moral development, with males emphasizing rules, while women focus on responsibility in relationships. Collier then explores the effect of these gender differences on the conduct of psychotherapy, both from the standpoint of the therapist and of the client. She is careful to point out that these differences are not absolute and advocates the need for each sex to learn from the other. Collier summarizes the qualities that her female self brings to the therapeutic process, and the paper ends with an exploration of the changing attitudes of males who seek psychotherapy.

In the next paper, "Family Therapy: A Field Guide," David Keith, starts with the hypothesis that many enter the profession of psychotherapy in an effort to deepen their connections with the self. However, too often professional training patterns take over and the self becomes dormant. The therapist may become prisoner of a model with damaging results for the patient. Indeed, for Keith, the dynamics of therapy are in the person of the therapist. If he cannot be a self, neither can the patient. Social change may take place, but there will be no gain in spontaneity. It is therefore essential that the therapist knows his "self" so that he may use it appropriately in therapy. Keith also points out that what applies to the self in family therapy does not automatically apply to individual therapy. Next, Keith discusses the difficulty in knowing the self. Relating his personal experience in dealing with the self, which is in fact a community of selves, he suggests that the term "familiarity" with the self is a more accurate descriptor than the term "knowledge" of the self. The paper then gives us glimpses of the self, collected over the last eight years, and describes manifestations of the self as it appears in therapy. He includes the issues of power, integrity, sense of the absurd and use of humor, freedom for anger and "creative hatred," metaphorical reality, the influence of outside experience, the development of peer relationships and the ability to let patients know that we love them. Keith concludes by stating that the patient's Self will only appear if invited by the therapist's Self.

In the last paper in this group of four, "Uses of the Self in Integrated Contextual Systems Therapy," Bunny Duhl explores the many ways in which she uses herself in therapy. She starts by giving a brief description of the family therapy model which was developed at the Boston Family Institute, a model which derives from general systems and learning theory. To facilitate change in such a model, the therapist helps people to internally update the way in which they hold beliefs, meanings and information and externally experience and enact alternative ways of behaving and relating. The task of the therapist is to tune people into their untapped resources and offer them tools with which to use these resources in daily life and problem solving. Duhl then briefly reviews the implication that such a model has for the training of therapists. The second half of the paper consists of relating problem-solving anecdotes from her own life which she has used successfully with her clients.

Whereas Bunny Duhl only alluded to her experience as a trainer of family therapists, the seventh paper in this collection by Harry J. Aponte and Joan E. Winter, "The Person and Practice of the Therapist: Treatment and Training," focuses on the development of the competency of the "person of the therapist." It starts by examining the four essential skills which a clinician needs in order to effect a positive therapeutic outcome in the authors' training model: external skills—technical behavior, in internal skills—integration of personal experience, theoretical and collaborative skills. They point out that although theoretical and collaborative skills are generally viewed as requisite for the clinical practitioner of any school of training, a major division exists between schools of training which focus on the technical and behavioral skills of the therapist—e.g., Haley and Minuchin—and those which stress the personal integration of the clinician—e.g., Bowen and Satir. Few programs offer an integration of both personal and technical skills. "The Person and Practice of the Therapist" training model does not depend on a specific clinical framework, and utilizes a generic teaching method which can accomodate a variety of clinical models. The theoretical framework in this approach is designed to elicit each participant's development of his own theories, technical and collaborative skills and how he uses himself as a person to attain positive outcomes with clients. Next, the authors contrast the psychoanalytic model of training, the "training analysis," with the Person-Practice model.

Whereas the counter-transference model refers only to the analyst's unconscious, the Person-Practice model draws primarily from the field of systems thinking and family therapy and incorporates every part of the system, the family, the therapist, as well as conscious and unconscious material. In order to operate in such a model, the therapist needs tremendous self-knowledge and discipline, hence the family therapist's need for personal work. The next section starts by pointing out how the therapist's personal life is often touched by the personal struggles of his clients. In the Person-Practice training model, the process of treatment acts as a potent stimulus to personal growth in which the therapist has an opportunity to deal with personal issues. After giving an overview of predominant models of training, the paper describes the goals, format and methods of the Person-Practice training model. The paper ends by illustrating the training process with a transcript of a training session and the trainee's written reaction to this intervention, followed by the transcript of a live therapy interview that the trainee conducted one month later.

The first of two papers concerned with research on the use of the self in family therapy is "The Effective Family Therapist: Some Old Data and

Some New Directions" by Alan S. Gurman, in which he reviews data on the personal qualities of the effective family therapist. He first examines five categories of characteristics which are independent of particular families, and points out that little research has been done to substantiate the importance of any of these variables in family therapy. His next step is to look at the process used by the effective family therapist during the actual conduct of treatment. After briefly reviewing the issue of the therapist's style and relationship skills, he points out that there is little conclusive research as to the impact of these two variables on the outcome of therapy. He also addresses the need to scrutinize whether or not there are therapist variables which are specific to family therapy.

Gurman suggests that such research is inconclusive because the right questions may not yet have been asked. He suggests that while there is probably a cluster of therapist characteristics that are minimal conditions for the effective practice of nearly all methods of family therapy, it is equally likely that different therapist "selves" may be required by different therapeutic schools. Gurman proposes to look at ways of conducting research in family therapy which may yield more definite results regarding the qualities of the effective family therapist. This will require researchers to have no vested interest in the outcome of their studies. In truth, the reason for choosing one method over another seems to be more related to personal factors than to the relative scientific status of one method versus another. He then posits that the way to ask the "right" questions is to convert the conviction of each approach to family therapy into more precise questions addressing issues which are specific to that particular approach. Gurman questions the appropriateness of applying traditional research designs to a circularly causal therapeutic system. He also cautions us about the limitations of linear as well as circular causality, one leading to meaningless reductionism and the other to useless generalities. In the search for understanding what an effective family therapist is and does, he advocates the need for combining "outcome" and "process" studies. He points out that such a process-outcome investigative model would be ecumenical and non-partisan, requiring that researchers know very clearly what they are trying to find out. They also need to be open to the possibility of finding out things they did not want to know!

Meri Shadley's participation in this collection came as part of a serendipitous experience in that by chance she made Michele Baldwin aware of her research on the professional development of family therapists. Since part of her research was focused on the use of self, we were delighted when she agreed to contribute to our project by authoring "Are all Therapists Alike? Use of Self in Family Therapy: A Multidimensional Perspective." Her purpose is to investigate how the therapist's use of self is viewed and approached across different schools of family therapy. The first theme which emerges from the data includes the therapist's definition and awareness of self. With slight variations, all interviewees agreed that professional and personal selves are intricately intertwined and that self awareness is critical to clinical effectiveness. Her second area of investigation deals with the critical aspects of therapeutic relationships. Most subjects indicated that the relationship skills of making connections, being warm and genuine, and providing encouragement and humor were important. Finally, Shadley examines the ways in which therapists utilized self-disclosure and, based on her findings, develops a continuum of self-disclosure styles. She reports specific differences in self-disclosure styles related primarily to gender and secondarily to clinical experience and theoretical orientation. The therapist's personal life experience also appears to be a factor in the therapist's use of self.

The collection ends with a paper which should put us at ease about our human frailties. In "Implications of the Wounded-Healer Paradigm for Use of the Self in Therapy," Grant Miller and DeWitt C. Baldwin explore the use of our wounded or vulnerable aspects to increase our professional effectiveness. For them, the helping relationship embodies the basic polarities inherent in the paradigm of the Wounded-Healer, polarities which ultimately relate to the vulnerabilities and healing power of both the healer and the patient. It is their belief that only through appropriate recognition and use of the helper's own vulnerability that healing power can effectively be realized in the therapeutic relationship. They start by giving a historical perspective on the concept of the wounded healer dating back to Greek mythology. They also provide a diagrammatic model to help analyze the interactional dynamics of the patient-healer encounter. They continue by describing the factors which facilitate healing. In addition to altruistic factors such as trust, warmth and empathy, conscious inner attention to oneself as a therapist must be present as well to be an effective healer. Such inner attention can be developed either in personal therapy during which unconscious elements emerge or are encouraged to be investigated, or through a conscious attention to one's sense of vulnerability emerging from the therapist's own pain and suffering. Miller and Baldwin assert that this makes possible an unconscious connection which activates the patient's healing power. In the process both experience a sense of wholeness. This paper concludes by suggesting that attention to one's vulnerabilities is not only indispensable to the healing process, but also decreases the likelihood of professional burn-out through the energizing experience of creativity by the therapist.

REFERENCES

Luft, J. & Ingham, H. (1963). *The Johari Window: A Graphic Model of Awareness in Interpersonal Relations*. Group Processes An Introduction to Group Dynamics. Palo Alto: National Press Books.
Luthman, S. G., & Kirschenbaum, M. (1974). *The Dynamic Family*. Palo Alto: Science and Behavior Books.

Rogers, Carl (In print). *A Client-Centered, Person-Centered Approach to Therapy.* In Psychotherapist's Casebook: Theory and Technique in Practice. I.L. Kutash and A. Wolf, Eds. San Francisco: Jossey-Bass.
Simon, R. (1986). *Our Quarterbacks and Coaches,* The Family Therapy Networker, March-April,
30-34.
Yalom, I.D. (1980). *Existential Psychotherapy,* New York: Basic Books, Inc.

The Therapist Story

Virginia Satir

ABSTRACT. Freud's contributions have radically altered our thinking about psychotherapy and human behavior. Although this has resulted in the development of many theories and techniques of therapy, the basic ingredient remains the relationship between the therapist and the patient. Since the latter comes to the former in a state of need, the therapist holds enormous power, which can be used negatively for exploitation and manipulation, or positively for healing and growth. The potential for the abuse of such power makes the value system and beliefs of the therapist vitally important. By being "congruent," the therapist can create a context of trust and caring, which enables the patient to dispell his or her fears and begin to explore new growth patterns. Therapy is a deeply intimate and vulnerable experience, requiring sensitivity to one's own state of being as well as to that of the other. It is the meeting of the deepest self of the therapist with the deepest self of the patient or client.

One hundred years ago, as today, we were nearing a new century. Then as now, people strongly felt that they lived in a period of great change. America was moving from a predominantly rural, agricultural way of life to an urban, industrial culture. The battle for human rights was emerging. Unions were forming to protect the rights of workers. Concerned citizens were lobbying for protection of children through child labor laws. Social reformers were mounting campaigns for women's suffrage. In the sciences, foundations were being laid for today's nuclear weaponry, space travel and electronic communications. In that same period, a new psychology was being formulated that would change the way we think about ourselves. I would like to think that the advent of another new century will bring with it another change of consciousness about ourselves—one that places a high value on humanness. The therapist who makes self an essential factor in the therapeutic process is a herald of that new consciousness.

Sigmund Freud opened his practice one hundred years ago in Vienna. In 1921, he visited the United States, bringing with him the new form of psychotherapy which he called psychoanalysis. His main thesis was that human beings carry the seeds of their construction as well as their

Virginia Satir, ACSW, is the Director of Training of the Avanta Network, 139 Forest Avenue, Palo Alto, CA 94301.

17

destruction within them. This was a radical idea that eventually initiated a revolutionary breakthrough in mental health practice. Up to that time, the prevailing reasons for deviant and other unacceptable forms of behavior were thought to be bad environment, personal unworthiness, and "genetic taint." The cure was usually isolation, punishment, abandonment, or death.

Freud's views also offered a new way of understanding human behavior. By 1940, psychoanalytic concepts underlay almost all psychological thinking and treatment and it continued that way until the appearance of existential and holistic thinking in the 60s. In some ways, I compare the impact of Freudian concepts with the work of Jellinek (1960), who advanced the idea that alcoholism was a disease and not the result of perversity or weakness. That, too, changed society's way of thinking and eventually led to new methods of treatment which offered hope to those who previously had no hope.

Originally, psychoanalytic treatment was administered by a trained psychotherapist (usually a physician) who, by "analyzing" the emotional experience and process of the patient, hoped to clear the way for the growth of health within the troubled individual. The early treatment model was that of the traditional doctor-patient relationship. The aim of treatment then, as it is today, was the eradication of symptoms, although the nature and meaning of symptoms have been greatly expanded over the years. The basic elements of psychotherapy remain the same, namely—a therapist, a patient, a context, the interaction between the therapist and patient, and a model for approaching treatment. However, the definitions of these elements have also expanded and changed through additions and deletions over time. For example, the "patient" now is sometimes known as the "client," and may represent an individual, a group or a family (Rogers, 1951). The therapist may also be called a counselor, and can include one, two, or even more persons. The therapist may be drawn from a variety of disciplines in addition to medicine and psychiatry, such as psychology, social work, education or theology. The context now includes the office, the home, the hospital, and the school.

The therapeutic interaction is also seen as a relationship between therapist and patient and may be characterized by a variety of treatment approaches, such as psychoanalysis, psychodrama, Gestalt therapy, transactional analysis, the various body therapies, family therapy and a host of others. The model of therapy has been expanded from the traditional, authoritarian doctor-patient relationship to include the patient as a partner (Hollender & Szasz, 1956).

We have all observed that two people using the same approach have come out with quite different results. We have also seen that two other people using quite different approaches can come out with similarly successful results. Yet very few training programs really deal with the person of the therapist. Those that do are usually in Psychoanalytic and Jungian Institutes where a training psychoanalysis is required or in some family training programs.

THE ROLE OF SELF IN THERAPY

Common sense dictates that the therapist and the patient must inevitably impact on one another as human beings. This involvement of the therapist's "self," or "personhood" occurs regardless of, and in addition to, the treatment philosophy or the approach. Techniques and approaches are tools. They come out differently in different hands. Because the nature of the relationship between therapist and patient makes the latter extremely vulnerable, it is encumbent upon the therapist to keep that relationship from being an exercise in the negative use of power, or of developing dependency, both of which ultimately defeat therapeutic ends.

Freud recognized the power of the therapist. He maintained that the successful therapist had to handle his personal life in such a way as not to become entangled in the personal life of the patient. This led to the neutral, non-personal format of the psychoanalytic couch, with the therapist out of sight and relatively non-active; this despite the fact that Freud is reported to have given massage at times to his patients and to have become actively involved in their lives. Needleman (1985) claims that the secret of Freud's great success and creativity was due to the great force of his personal attention to his patients, which enabled him to project a quality of compassion and insight which radiated a healing influence.

Perhaps doubting his own capacity and that of others not to negatively influence pateints, Freud developed the idea of mandatory training analysis for all psychotherapists, during which the trainees were supposed to understand and master their own conflicts and neuroses. This requirement was aimed at protecting the patient and creating the optimum conditions for change.

These ideas clearly stood on two basic principles: That therapists have the power to damage patients, and they are there to serve patients, not the other way around. Most therapists today would agree that they would not consciously want to harm their patients. On the contrary, they would claim that they try to create treatment contexts that are beneficial to their patients. Most therapists would also say that they are there to serve their patients. However, the words "harm" and "serve" are open to many interpretations.

Furthermore, there was, and is, the idea that unconsciously, without malice or intent, therapists can harm patients through their own unresolved problems (Langs, 1985). One manifestation is reflected in what Freud called counter-transference. Briefly, this means that therapists mistakenly and unconsciously see patients as a sons, daughters, mothers or fathers, thereby projecting onto their patients something which does not belong—a real case of mistaken identity. This is a trap, well recognized by many therapists. However, unless therapists are very clear and aware, they may be caught in the trap without knowing it. Unless one knows what is going on, it is tempting to blame the patient for a feeling of being "stuck" as a therapist. A further manifestation of this phenomenon is rescuing or protecting, taking sides, or rejecting a patient, and, again, putting the responsibility on the patient.

When the prevailing model of therapeutic transaction, the authoritarian doctor-patient relationship, is experienced as one of dominance and submission, the patient and therapist can easily move into a power play which tends to reinforce childhood learning experiences. Throughout the therapeutic experience, the therapist may unwittingly replicate the negative learning experiences of the patient's childhood and call it treatment. For instance, when a therapist maintains that she knows when she doesn't know, she is modelling behavior similar to that of the patient's parent. The dominance and submission model increases chances for the therapist to live out her own ego needs for control. Manifestations of this control can appear to be benevolent, as in "I am the one who helps you; therefore, you should be grateful," or malevolent, as in "you'd better do what I tell you, or I won't treat you." These, of course, are shades of childhood past. When they are present in therapy, treatment aims will be defeated.

POWER AND THERAPY

The above are all disguised power issues. But, power has two faces: one, is controlling the other; the second is empowering the other. The use of power is a function of the self of the therapist. It is related to the therapist's self-worth, which governs the way in which the therapist handles her ego needs. Use of power is quite independent of any therapeutic technique or approach, although there are some therapeutic approaches which actually are based on the therapist maintaining a superior position (Dreikurs, 1960). There also are cases where there is outright and conscious exploitation by the therapist and some even justify their aggresive, sexual, or other unprofessional behavior on the grounds that it is beneficial to the patient (Langs, 1985). Once, a man came to my office with a bullwhip in his hand and asked me to beat him with it so he could become sexually potent. While I believed that it was possible that his method would work for him, I rejected it on the basis that it did not fit my values. I offered to help him in other ways and he accepted.

Using patients for one's own ego needs or getting them mixed up with one's own life is ethically unsound. However, the therapist can be in the same position as the patient, denying, distorting or projecting needs. It is possible for a patient or a client to activate something within the therapist of which the latter is unaware. It is easy to respond to a patient as though he or she is someone else in one's past or present, and if one is not aware that this going on it will needlessly complicate the situation. If one is a family therapist, it is likely that somewhere, at least once, one will see a family that duplicates some aspects of one's own family. When this happens and the therapist has not yet worked out the difficulties with his or her own family, the client may be stranded or misled because the therapist also is lost. Therapists should recognize that they are just as vulnerable as patients.

While therapists facilitate and enhance patients' ability and need to grow, they should at the same time be aware that they have the same ability and need. One way to avoid "burn-out" is to keep growing and learning. A great part of our behavior is learned from modeling and therapists can model ways of learning and growing. It is also important to model congruence. An over-simplified definition of congruence is that one looks like one feels, says what one feels and means and acts in accordance with what one says. Such congruence develops trust. This is the basis for the emotional honesty between therapist and patient which is the key to healing. When a therapist says one thing and feels another, or demonstrates something that she denies, she is creating an atmosphere of emotional dishonesty which makes it an unsafe environment for the patient. I find that there is a level of communication beyond words and feelings, in which life communicates with life and understands incongruence. Young children show this awareness more easily. In adults, this level of communication usually presents itself in hunches or in vague feelings of uneasiness, or sensing. If I, as a therapist, am denying, distorting, projecting or engaging in any other form of masking, and am unaware of my own inner stirrings, I am communicating these to those around me no matter how well I think I am disguising them.

If patients feel that they are at risk because they feel "one down" in relation to the therapist, they will not report their distressed feelings and will develop defenses against the therapist. The therapist in turn, not knowing about this, can easily misunderstand the patient's response as resistance, instead of legitimate self-protection against the therapist's incongruence. Therapy is an intimate experience. For people to grow and change they need to be able to allow themselves to become open, which makes them vulnerable. When they are vulnerable, they need protection. It is the therapist's responsibility to create a context in which people feel and are safe, and this requires sensitivity to one's own state. For example, it is quite possible for a therapist who is focusing on a technique or a theoretical construct to be unaware that her own facial features and voice tone are conveying the messages to which the patient is responding.

The presence of resistance is a manifestation of fear and calls for the utmost in honesty, congruence and trust on the part of the therapist. The only times that I have experienced difficulty with people are when I was incongruent. I either tried to be something I wasn't, or to withhold something I knew, or to say something I did not mean. I have great respect for that deep level of communication where one really knows when and whom one can trust. I think it comes close to what Martin Buber called the "I-Thou" relationship. (Buber, 1970).

Very little change goes on without the patient and therapist becoming vulnerable. Therapists know that they have to go beyond patient defenses, so they can help them to become more open and vulnerable. Defenses are ways patients try to protect themselves when they feel unsafe. When the therapist acts to break down defenses, the therapeutic interaction becomes an experience which is characterized by "Who has the right to tell whom what to do, or who wins." In this struggle, the therapist, like the parent, has to win and the patient loses.

When the patient is somehow thought of as a trophy on the therapist's success ladder, this is another repetition of the way in which many children experience their parents—where they were expected to be a show case for family values. Sometimes the therapist puts the patient in a position of being a pawn between two opposing authorities—as when a therapist puts a child between the parents, or between the parents and an institutional staff.

When the therapist sets out to help someone and leaves no doubt that she knows what is best for the patient, she is subjecting the patient to repetition of another childhood experience. There are those therapists who feel challenged to make something of the patient, "even if it kills you." These are often therapists who want to give messages of validation, although the outcomes are often very different.

THE POSITIVE USE OF THE SELF

If the therapist can influence therapeutic results negatively through their use of self, then it must be possible to use the self for positive results. The therapist has that power by virtue of her role and status and person. We know that this power can be misused and misdirected. However, the therapist also has the choice to use her power for empowering. Because the patient is vulnerable, the therapist can use her power to empower patients towards their own growth.

In the new model of treatment that emerged in the 1950s and 1960s, the therapist began to form a partnership with the patient. Patient and therapist could work together utilizing their respective actions, reactions, and interactions. The therapist was encouraged to model congruent behavior, and the focus of the therapeutic partnership was on developing health through working with the whole person. Eradication of the symptom was achieved by the development of a healthy state, which no longer required the symptom. In the traditional, authoritarian doctor-patient model, the emphasis was first on eradicating the symptom, with the hope that health would follow.

When the emphasis is totally on empowering the patient, the therapist will tend to choose methods that serve that purpose. When therapists work at empowering, the patient is more likely to have opportunities to experience old attitudes in new contexts. (Rogers, 1961a, 1980). They have the experience of literally interacting with their therapists, of getting and giving feedback. The treatment context becomes a life-learning and life-giving context between the patient and a therapist, who responds personally and humanly. The therapist is clearly identified as a self interacting with another self. Within this context the therapist's use of self is the main tool for change. Using self, the therapist builds trust and rapport so more risks can be taken. Use of the self by the therapist is an integral part of the therapeutic process and it should be used consciously for treatment purposes.

MY USE OF MY SELF

I have learned that when I am fully present with the patient or family, I can move therapeutically with much greater ease. I can simultaneously reach the depths to which I need to go, and at the same time honor the fragility, the power and the sacredness of life in the other. When I am in touch with myself, my feelings, my thoughts, with what I see and hear, I am growing toward becoming a more integrated self. I am more congruent, I am more "whole," and I am able to make greater contact with the other person. When I have spoken of these concepts in workshops, people thank me for speaking out, legitimizing what they have been feeling themselves. In a nutshell, what I have been describing are therapists who put their personhood and that of their patients first. It is the positive people-contact which paves the way for the risks that have to be taken. Many adults have reported they did not feel they were in contact with their parents and the others who brought them up. They did not feel like persons, but were treated as roles or expectations. If the therapeutic situation cannot bring out the people contact, then what chance does it have for really making it possible for people to feel differently themselves?

The metaphor of a musical instrument comes to mind when I think of the therapist's use of the self. How it is made, how it is cared for, its fine tuning and the ability, experience, sensitivity and creativity of the player will determine how the music will sound. Neither the player nor the instrument writes the music. A competent player with a fine instrument can play well almost any music designed for that instrument. An incompetent player with an out-of-tune instrument will vilify any music, indicating that the player has an insensitive, untrained ear. I think of the instrument as the self of the therapist: how complete one is as a person, how well one cares for oneself, how well one is tuned in to oneself, and how competent one is at one's craft. I think of the music as the presentation of the patient. How that music is heard and understood by the therapist is a large factor in determining the outcome of the therapy.

I give myself permission to be totally clear and in touch with myself. I also give myself full permission to share my views, as well as permission to see if my views have validity for the people with whom I am working. The person of the therapist is the center point around which successful therapy revolves. The theories and techniques are important. I have developed many of them. But, I see them as tools to be used in a fully human context. I further believe that therapists are responsible for the initiation and continuation of the therapy process. They are not in charge of the patients within that process.

The whole therapeutic process must be aimed at opening up the healing potential within the patient or client. Nothing really changes until that healing potential is opened. The way is through the meeting of the deepest self of the therapist with the deepest self of the person, patient or client. When this occurs, it creates a context of vulnerability—of openness to change.

This clearly brings in the spiritual dimension. People already have what they need to grow and the therapist's task is to enable patients to utilize their own resources. If I believe that human beings are sacred, then when I look at their behavior, I will attempt to help them to live up to their own sacredness. If I believe that human beings are things to be manipulated, then I will develop ways to manipulate them. If I believe that patients are victims, then I will try to rescue them. In other words, there is a close relationship between what I believe and how I act. The more in touch I am with my beliefs, and acknowledge them, the more I give myself freedom to choose how to use those beliefs.

What started as a radical idea 100 years ago has become part of a recognized psychology predicted upon the belief that human beings have capacity for their own growth and healing. In this century, there has been more research and attention given to the nature of the human being than ever before. As we approach the 21st century, we know a great deal about how the body and brain work and how we learn. We can transplant organs, we can create artificial intelligence, we can go to the moon and other planets. We can communicate anywhere in the world instantly by satellite. We can fly across the Atlantic in three hours—a trip that took several weeks, 100 years ago. We have also created the biggest monster of all time—the nuclear bomb. We still haven't learned to accept a positive way of dealing with conflict.

Amid these changes is the growing conviction that human beings must evolve a new consciousness that places a high value on being human, that leads toward cooperation, that enables positive conflict resolution and that recognizes our spiritual foundations. Can we accept as a given that the self of the therapist is an essential factor in the therapeutic process? If this turns out to be true, it will alter our way of teaching therapists as well as treating patients.

We started out knowing that the person of the therapist could be harmful to the patient. We concentrated on ways to avoid that. Now, we need to concentrate on ways in which the use of self can be of positive value in treatment.

REFERENCES

Buber, M., (1970). *I and Thou*. New York: Charles Scribners.

Dreikurs, R., (1960). The Current Dilemma in Psychotherapy. *J. Exist. Psych.* 1:187.

Freud, S., (1959). *Collected Papers*. Vol. II. New York: Basic Books.

Hollender, M.H. & Szasz, T.S. (1956). A Contribution to the Philosophy of Medicine, *Arch. Intern. Med.* 97:585-592.

Jellinek, E.M., (1960). *The Disease Concept of Alcoholism*. New Haven: College and University Press.

Langs, R. (1985). *Madness and Cure*. Emerson, NJ: Newconcept Press.

Maslow, A. (1962). *Toward a Psychology of Being*. 2nd Ed., New York: Van Nostrand Reinhold.

Needleman, J. (1985). *The Way of the Physician*. New York: Harper and Row.

Rogers, C. (1951). *Client-Centered Therapy*. Boston: Houghton-Mifflin.

Rogers, C. (1961a). *The Process Equation of Psychotherapy*. Am . J. *Psychotherapy* 15:27-45.

Rogers, C. (1961b). *On Becoming a Person*. Boston: Houghton-Mifflin.

Yalom, I. (1980). *Existential Psychotherapy*. New York: Basic Books.

Some Philosophical
and Psychological Contributions
to the Use of Self in Therapy

DeWitt C. Baldwin, Jr.

ABSTRACT. The question of why the concept of the use of self in therapy should emerge at this time is discussed, together with its philosophical and psychological antecedents. The article's thesis is that while the idea of the self has fascinated man throughout history, it was Kierkegaard and the existential philosophers who persuasively shifted attention from the essence of man to the nature of his existence and the world of subjective experience. This permitted the emergence of a self which was not merely a product of instinctual drives or of external forces, but was an interacting being, which could be both subject and object at the same time. Major figures in this development include philosophers such as Heidegger, writers such as Sartre, clinicians such as Carl Rogers, sociologists such as George Herbert Mead, and theologians such as Tillich. Buber's insightful elaboration of the "I-Thou" relationship is felt to be a landmark contribution, underlying many recent developments in humanistic psychology and psychotherapy. The concept of the use of self in therapy, then, is seen as standing in unique relation to confluent streams of thought from the fields of existential philosophy, phenomenology, psychiatry, psychotherapy, personality development, symbolic interactionism and humanistic psychology.

INTRODUCTION

It is always interesting to speculate why certain ideas emerge at a particular time. It is especially intriguing to review the reasons why attention should be called at this time to the use of self in therapy. According to systems theory, the therapist is unavoidably part of the treatment situation, both as therapist (change agent) and as himself. He does not choose to be in or out, he can only choose to be aware or not. That this role can operate along a continuum from activity to passivity has been alluded to by a number of authors (Hollender & Szasz, 1956). Indeed, a major development of the past several decades has been the increasingly active and

---

DeWitt C. Baldwin, Jr., M.D., is currently Director of Education Research at the American Medical Association, 535 North Dearborn St., Chicago, IL 60610, and Adjunct Professor of Health Professions Education at the Center for Educational Development, the University of Illinois at Chicago. He previously served as President of Earlham College.

participatory role in such transactions accorded to the patient (Fink, 1979). In this particular evolution, the seminal work of Carl Rogers must be noted, in that he saw the potential for self-direction in patients, whom he began to refer to as "clients," viewing the therapist as assisting rather than promoting the process of self-determination and development.

It is not surprising that the movement towards a more humanistic psychology which emerged after World War II was accepted by many therapists, who found the determinism and reductionism of the Freudian view unsatisfactory from a personal and professional standpoint. This resulted in an outpouring of interest in the uniqueness and authenticity of human experience. Belief in the self-actualizing ability of man led to the formation of the human potential movement of the 1960s and 70s (Maslow, 1962). Unfortunately, proponents of this movement often carried the idea of personal growth to the limits of personal license and failed to develop a disciplined and systematic examination of its assumptions and implications. Each person's experience was considered valid in itself and, in the place of the rigidities of traditional psychiatry and psychology, there emerged a plethora of therapeutic systems and approaches, based on individual style, inclination and popularity. Indeed, the field of therapy appeared to move from an excessive dependence upon rigid theories and formats to an equally excessive emphasis on idiosyncratic techniques and therapeutic stratagems, which, often as not, were more artificial and manipulative than the traditional approaches.

Recent attempts to bring order out of such confusion have been based on the finding that the differences between patients/clients treated with different approaches and techniques tend to be rather minimal (Wolpe, 1961; Strupp, 1963, 1973). Yalom (1980) cites research which attempted to correlate client and therapist perceptions of key moments of change or growth in therapy, only to find that what the therapist imagined was critical or insightful was frequently not so perceived by the client or patient (Standal & Corsini, 1959). Indeed, there is increasing acceptance among therapists of all persuasions that there is something in the unique nature of the therapeutic relationship and the person of the therapist which plays a critical role in the process of therapy (Rogers, 1961a, 1961c, 1986; Truax et al., 1966a, 1966b). Since this awareness comes close to what Martin Buber (1923) referred to in the early part of the century as the essential quality of the "I-Thou" relationship, a brief look at a definition of the self and at some of the philosophical and psychological developments which have contributed to this concept is in order.

THE CONCEPT OF THE SELF

The nature of the self has intrigued writers and philosophers throughout the ages. Its very definition comes close to overwhelming the Oxford English Dictionary, with some five pages devoted to attempting to define the word itself in its many senses and forms, and another 14 pages to its many modifications.

For the ancients, the idea of self was usually implicit in the concept of the soul, which was conceived of as the vital, immaterial, life-principle, or "essence" of man (Roccatagliata, 1986). Primitive religions saw the soul as directing or controlling both mental and physical processes in man. The cessation of these, as in death, inevitably posed the unanswerable question of immortality—a question which has occupied a central place in all subsequent religious thought. While Hinduism and Buddhism do not admit the existence of the individual soul, the doctrine of reincarnation provides a vehicle for man to obtain progressively higher levels of virtue and piety. For Islam and later Judaism, the soul comes from God and, thus, is independent of the body; but, for the pious, it is rejoined with the body on the Day of Judgement. Influenced by the neo-Platonists, many medieval and later Christians believed that the God-given soul existed in a dualistic relation with an inferior and earth-bound body.

The nature of the soul also has intrigued philosophers. Plato believed in the immortality of the soul, which he saw as separate and distinct from the body, from which it was released by death for full expression. Aristotle began as a Platonist, viewing the soul as immaterial, but in "De Anima" (On the Soul) he later described the soul as the inseparable, substantial form of the living organism, guiding and directing it. He further defined the soul in terms of vegetative, animal and rational functions, thereby setting the stage for later preoccupation with the mind/body relationship.

This view reached its acme in Descartes' famous statement "cogito, ergo sum" (I think, therefore, I am), and the subsequent dualism of body and mind with which he is identified. This position, of course, served to draw the battlelines between a concern with the external, objective, natural world of objects and the less accessible, more subjective, inner world. Despite its limitations, and the criticisms currently directed toward Cartesian dualism by biobehavioral research, this concept enabled the development of critical inquiry in the physical sciences in a way that has made possible much of today's progress in science and technology. Because of this emphasis, however, the objective and materialistic side of life achieved a commanding lead over that of the subjective and non-conscious, and it was not until philosophers such as Kierkegaard and Husserl, writers such as Dostoevski and Tolstoy, and clinicians such as Freud, Jung and Adler, that the subjective world began to be explored in terms more appropriate to its understanding.

Freud's theories initiated a renewed attack upon the established lines of Cartesian dualism by adding the elusive concept of the unconscious to confuse the comfortable physical terms to which the domain of the mental and conscious had been assigned. In his 1915 paper on "The Unconscious," Freud (1934) differentiated between unconscious ideas, which continue to exist as formations after repression, and unconscious affects, which are discharged. He and his followers went on to describe a whole continuum of the unconscious, from lack of awareness of vegetative and neurological processes to fantasy and dreams. While his emphasis on psychic determinism confused the philosophers, it served to stimulate a new and fruitful discussion of the concept of the self, both among his followers and those in other disciplines. At the same time, it must be remembered that Freud basically was a scientist and did not, himself, directly challenge the heavy investment which science had in Cartesian dualism. Thus, despite the efforts of William James, John Dewey and others to examine the self on an empirical basis, the concept of a self, complete with philosophical, social and religious connotations, was largely ignored by an emerging psychology seeking to establish itself as a scientific discipline.

It was the writers and philosophers, primarily from the existential school, who continued to explore the world of subjective phenomenology. Still, it remained for George Herbert Mead (1934) to reintroduce the concept of the self as a basic unit of personality into scientific thought, along with the roles which the self learns to take in the course of its socialization. He saw the self as a process rather than a structure, and maintained that self and the consciousness of self emerged from social interaction—the interaction of the human organism with its social environment. He believed that what made man unique was his capacity to be both subject and object at the same time. Since he could even be an object of his own thought and action, self-interaction, he stood in a markedly different relation to his environment than the then prevailing view of behavior as resulting from external factors or internal drives. His work, while not theoretically explicit, laid the groundwork for the later development of symbolic interactionism, a field that has greatly influenced modern sociological and psychological thought. Indeed, the revival of interest in the self has been so widespread that it is difficult to find a modern personality theory that does not place the self in a central position (Arieti, 1967; Kohut, 1971, 1985).

Special note must be made of the contributions of the developmentalists, such as Erikson and Greenacre, who described the emerging self in terms of the psychosexual and ego-development of the child. They noted the fundamental absence of a distinction between the self and the not-self as basic characteristics of the newborn, who, partly as a result of his perceptions, begins to differentiate various aspects of his body image from objects in the external world. Multiple self-presentations gradually lead to the formation of a concept of the self, which becomes more stable and permanent as a result of the achievement of object constancy.

Closely related is the concept of identity (Greenacre, 1958; Erikson, 1950, 1959), which constitutes an awareness of separateness and distinction from all others, in which the borders of the self are hypercathected by the early experience of separation from the mother. Thus, the distinction of the "I" from the "not-I" is reinforced by a variety of internal and external experiences. Indeed, the mechanism of projection is based on the primal lack of distinction between the self and the not-self. These contributions have allowed Speigel (1959) to define the self "as a frame of reference or zero point to which representations of specific mental and physical states are referred and against which they are perceived and judged."

It is clear, however, that Cartesian dualism still plays an influential role in modern life and thought. As Buber (1955, 1965, 1970) points out, most of our transactions with our fellow man and our environment are in the nature of subject-object, or I-It relationships. In calling attention to man's essential need to participate in reciprocal I-Thou relationships, in which each person fully regards and accepts the subject and object both in self and other, Buber pleads for a reunification of man's subjective and objective parts. Far from being merely the absence of an infantile distinction between the subjective and objective, or the self and not-self, this is the achievement of a new unity which, while existing in both conscious and unconscious spheres, is available and accessible to the dedicated searcher.

The use of self in therapy, then, as a subject of theoretical and practical psychotherapeutic importance, emerges at this time in history, largely because of the re-emergence of a concern with the uniqueness of human experience and relationship over the past century.

THE CONTRIBUTIONS OF EXISTENTIAL PHILOSOPHY

Perhaps the most important influence on the 20th century view of man and on the emerging concept of the use of self in therapy comes from the existential philosophers, who take their lead from the seminal work of Soren Kierkegaard (1959). Writing out of the depths of his own personal concerns, Kierkegaard objected to Hegel's efforts to unite the ambiguities of life in an abstract fashion through positing of a higher synthesis. He insisted that the dichotomies of life—good and evil, life and death, God and man—could not be mediated, but that man was called upon to make decisions between these polarities. He asked man to turn from the world of thought to that of existence as it is actually lived, believing that only through an examination of human experience in all its complexity could one approach the basic question: "What is the meaning of life?"

Kierkegaard believed that meaning is to be found in the decisions between such polarities and that these decisions must be based on one's own closely examined experience, rather than on any authority or abstract concept. Such an act, of course, is frightening, in that one is asked to abandon the usual sources of support and to leap into the unknown. It was his belief that each individual must, of necessity, make fully conscious, responsible choices among the alternatives that life offers. His works, "Sickness Unto Death" and "The Concept of Dread," are classics of early depth psychology. The former alludes to the role of the unconscious in depression, while the latter makes a clear distinction between "angst" (dread), which he defines as a feeling that has no definite object, and the fear and terror that derive from an objective threat.

It was not until some time after his death that the philosophical and psychological implications of Kierkegaard's work began to be fully appreciated. Indeed, existentialism is generally viewed as a 20th century phenomenon and has profoundly affected the development of philosophy, religion and psychology in this century. Within this century, seminal thinkers in the development of existentialism have included the religious thinkers Bultmann, Marcel and Tillich, as well as those who have clearly disassociated themselves from the religious view, such as Sartre and Camus. Of note in this development is the work of Edmund Husserl (1965), who introduced the phenomenological method in philosophy, calling upon man to examine his own experience. Of special importance was his insistence on "intentionality," the idea that every meaningful world must be rooted in the experience of which it is only a name, stating "Consciousness is always consciousness of something."

While rejecting the existential label, Heidegger (1962) is usually regarded as the figurehead of 20th century existentialism. He believed that we can learn something about the fundamental nature of man—his "being-in-the-world"—through an analysis of his anxieties, particularly, his fear of death. He accepted life as fundamentally contingent, stating that the only way to live authentically is to accept our own finitude and to develop a capacity to care (Sorge). This includes not just "solicitude" for others, as suggested by the later existential psychologists, but also an ontological caring for, or custodianship, of Being.

Tillich (1952) differed from Heidegger in believing that it is in "the boundary situation"—that situation in which one is denied the supports of authority and intellectualism, and even the traditional concept of God is found wanting—that one finds the unconditional certainty of the "Ground of Being," the "Being—itself," which appears when all else has been dissolved in anxiety and doubt. He believed that we are all aware of the contrast between the ideals which we hold and the lives we live, calling this the difference between "essence" and "existence." He maintained that we can resolve this difference only in the "boundary situation," defining authenticity as "the courage to be" and, thus, to escape "non-being."

Perhaps the most radical of the modern existentialists was Jean Paul Sartre (1950). He concluded that man is not only "en-soi" (in himself)—a passive recipient of fate—but also "pour-soi" (for himself), transcending the present. Thus, he is free from the limitations imposed by the world of experience. Indeed, he is forced to be free. To live authentically means to accept this dreadful freedom and to see that values are merely projections of his decisions. Such a position suggests a radical nihilism and individualism, which has strongly influenced the development of the field.

THE INFLUENCE OF MARTIN BUBER

Although he rejected the label during his lifetime, Buber's thought was profoundly influenced by existentialism (1923, 1955, 1965, 1970). He believed that man's access to being is neither through the ideal forms of Plato, nor through the "existent" as in Heidegger, but, rather, through man's capacity to enter into dialogue or relationship with the existent, or "the between." He rejected the traditional idea of reason as the distinctive characteristic of man, but, rather, defined him as a "creature capable of entering into living relation with the world and things, with men both as individuals and as the many, and with the 'mystery of being'—which is dimly apparent through all this but infinitely transcends it" (Friedman, 1965, p. 16). Thus, man is unique in his capacity to participate in both finitude and infinity. Man, Buber states, is "the crystallized potentiality of existence."

Starting from a concern with man's three vital relationships, those between God and man, man and man, and man and nature, Buber's views were elaborated in "Ich und Du" (1923), in which he states that man's relation to God, the Great Thou, enables him to participate in I-Thou relationships with other humans. For Buber, I-Thou "establishes the world of relation," into which both parties enter in the fullness of their being, with a sense of and appreciation for the subject and object in each. It is a relationship "characterized by mutuality, directness, presentness, intensity, and ineffability" (Friedman, 1965, p. 12).

This is contrasted with the I-It, or subject-object, relationship, in which others are regarded as mere tools or conveniences. I-It is the medium of exchange in the world of things and ideas, dealing with categories and connections, with experiencing and using. Indeed, the scientific method is man's most highly perfected development of the I-It, or subject-object, way of knowing. It is qualified to compare object with object, even man with man, but not to know his wholeness or his uniqueness.

The I-Thou relationship, on the other hand, is immediate and unmediated. There is no intervening purpose. It is an end and not a means. It is enduring—"always there in potentiality, waiting to be touched— released, known" It is not fixed in time or space. It is only in the now—the moment. However, he warns, "one cannot live in the pure present: it would consume us" (Buber, 1970, p. 85).

It also is responsibility—in the sense of one's response to another. "There is a reciprocity of giving: you say You to it and give yourself to it; it says You to you and gives itself to you" (ibid., p. 84). It is through this relation that man becomes known to himself and to others as a self. "Man becomes an I through a You" (ibid., p. 80). Self-realization, thus, is the by-product, rather than the goal, as is often assumed.

For Buber, the highest expression of the I-Thou relationship lies in the act of confirming the other. He sees mutual confirmation as the key element in the definition of the self. Man realizes his uniqueness only in relation to another who reciprocally defines himself. Each becomes confirmed by the other in his true, real, present, authentic self. Indeed, he states, so great is man's need for such definition and confirmation that he would rather be falsely confirmed than not confirmed at all—an act of "seeming," rather than "being." True confirmation is mutual and involves making the other fully present in all his unity and uniqueness.

Buber on Psychotherapy

In a unique dialogue which took place between Martin Buber and Carl Rogers in 1957 (Friedman, 1965), Buber drew a distinction between acceptance, or affirmation of the other, as emphasized by Rogers ("what one is"), and confirmation, which not only accepts, but actively engages the polarity in the other, including his potential for the worst within, by helping him against himself ("what one can become"). He further distinguished between the I-Thou relationship and that of therapist-patient, by stating that the helping relationship is necessarily one-sided. The two persons involved are not truly equal, in that the patient expects something from the therapist and the latter accepts that responsibility. Buber maintains that the goal of psychotherapy is the healing of the patient and the relation to that goal inevitably differs between therapist and patient. Furthermore, what is explored in therapy is the patient's experience, not that of the therapist. In other words, while the therapist can empathize and extend himself into the world of the patient, the reverse is not usually the case. The patient cannot experience the relationship from the side of the therapist without fundamentally altering or destroying it.

Buber describes true dialogue as that occurring "between partners who have turned to one another in truth, who express themselves without reserve and are free of the desire for semblance" (Buber, 1965, p. 86), where neither one is ruled by the thought of his effect on the other. He maintains that even the most genuine and authentic of therapeutic relationships cannot permit the awareness of consciousness on the part of the therapist that he understands or experiences a greater reality than that of the client. This is not to say that an accepting, positive regard and genuine concern for the full potentialities of the patient on the part of the therapist cannot lead to confirmation and "healing" (wholeness), but that this, in Buber's mind, is not really a genuine dialogue between equals with equal perceptions of each other's experience and of the situation.

For Buber, genuine dialogue cannot be arranged in advance, and is granted rather than created. The essential quality of therapy is authentic presence—not just being present, although that is necessary. Nor is it merely being in the present—that, too, is necessary. What is unique is the quality of presence—of being totally available, in tune with the other, without boundary, without limit. Thus, he goes beyond Rogers' acceptance and "unconditional, positive regard," and Heidegger's solicitude or caring (Sorge) for others, in advocating the offer of one's "total being" to another. Incidentally, it is important to realize that Buber intended his relational concepts to apply to the realities of community living, as well (the essential "WE"), a point of considerable relevance for group and family therapy.

In the same year, the Washington School of Psychiatry invited Buber to give the William Alanson White Memorial Lectures, along with a series of seminars. In speaking of psychotherapy, Buber stated "I have the impression (that) more and more therapists are not so confident that this or that theory is right and have (developed) a more "musical" floating relationship to their patients. The deciding reality is the therapist, not the methods" (quoted in Friedman, 1965, p. 37). At another point, he states: "There are two kinds of therapists: One who knows more or less consciously the kind of interpretation of dreams he will get; and the other . . . . who does not know. I am entirely on the side of the latter, who does not want something precise. He is ready to receive what he will receive. He cannot know what method he will use beforehand. He is, so to speak, in the hands of his patient" (ibid., p. 37). In other words, he must be ready to be surprised. "It is much easier to impose oneself on the patient than it is to use the whole force of one's soul to leave the patient to himself and not to touch him. The real master responds to uniqueness" (ibid., p. 38).

THE CONCEPT OF THE SELF
IN PSYCHOANALYSIS AND PSYCHIATRY

Otto Kernberg (1974) points out that "psychoanalytic theory has always included the concept of the self, that is, the individual's integrated conception of himself, as an experiencing, thinking, valuing and acting (or interacting) entity. . . . In fact, Freud's starting point in describing the "I" ("Das ich," so fatefully translated as "the ego" in English) was that of the conscious person whose entire intrapsychic life was powerfully influenced by dynamic, unconscious forces.'' At the same time, it is clear that Freud's focus on building instinctual and structural theories led to difficulties with integrating a broad concept of the self which spoke to its many dimensions. Jung was undoubtedly aware of this problem when he wrote ''as an empirical concept, the self designates the whole range of psychic phenomena in man. It expresses the unity of the personality as a whole'' (Jung, 1971, pp. 425, 460). He saw the ultimate outcome of the process of individuation as ''the realization of the self.'' This focus on the self, of course, was ultimately based on the assumption of most psycho-dynamically-oriented schools that if you changed the inner self of the patient, behavioral changes would follow, a view held in the reverse by the behaviorists. It is also important to note that until relatively recently, this focus was entirely on the self of the patient and did not expressly involve the use of the therapist's own self in the therapeutic process.

It remained for the Neo-Freudians, Sullivan, Horney and others, to more fully develop and integrate the concept of the self into their theories and practice. Sullivan (1953) refers to the self-system as the central dynamism of human organization, describing dynamism as ''the relatively enduring patterns of energy transformation, which recurrently characterize the interpersonal relations . . . which make the distinctively human sort of being.'' He states that personifications of the ''good me'' and the ''bad me,'' reflected through the appraisals of significant adults, leads to awareness of a sense of ''not me,'' which is overwhelmingly anxiety-producing. He believes that the feeling of self-esteem, which is based on the interplay between these, is essential to healthy functioning and to an understanding of mental illness. One of his major contributions was to see therapy as an interpersonal process, requiring active participation by the therapist. Since the latter's values, feelings and attitudes are part of this process, counter-transference becomes an important consideration.

Horney (1939, 1950) also felt that libido theory and its derived postulates did not adequately explain her clinical observations. She decided that the nuclear conflict of neurosis was not one of instincts, but of self-attitudes. She views the self as the dynamic core of human personality, ''the central inner force, common to all human beings, and yet unique in each, which is the deep source of (healthy) growth'' (1950, p. 17). She sees the self as the source of our capacities for experiencing and expressing feelings, for evolving values and making choices, and for taking responsibility for our actions. She, too, believes that self-esteem represents the healthy development of appropriate self-attitudes, based on real and genuine capacities, rather than illusions or self-deceptions. She held a central belief ''in the inner dignity and freedom of man and the constructiveness of evolutionary forces inherent in man.''

Heinz Kohut (1971, 1985), likewise, eschews drive theory for a more encompassing focus on the concept of the self in his comprehensive theory of the development of the self and the treatment of its disorders. While his views have evolved over time, he regards narcissism and object love—love of self and love of the other—as two separate but intertwined lines of development, each of which is essential to our ability to function and to love. More relevant to this paper is his insistence on the gathering of primary data from empathetic observation of the patient's inner-experience, and a shift in the role of the therapist toward maintaining an empathetic, rather than objective stance. He believes that it is the therapist's task to place himself "in the skin" of the patient and to understand what each situation feels like to that patient. This enables the therapist to create a supportive framework, which serves to replace the missing elements in the primary mother/child relationship, and both provides and models a "corrective emotional experience," which enables the patient to rediscover his unique developmental path. He believes that introspection and empathy are essential components of psychoanalytic fact-finding and are key elements in the therapist's relationship to his patient.

The concept of the self likewise holds an important place in the writings of Silvano Arieti (1967) and the Cognitive-Volitional School. Their emphasis, however, is on the symbolic and volitional mechanisms by which the self is defined in its relations with others in the outside world. In addition, they are concerned with the sequence of external influences and the intrapsychic mechanisms by which these influences are integrated into that part of the human psyche that in various terminologies has been called the "inner or intrapsychic self." By this very statement, however, Arieti appears to identify the self as some part or substrate of the person, rather than the totality posited by Buber and others. Indeed, Arieti elaborates the existence of a primordial or presymbolic self, a primary self and a secondary self as stages in development tied to cognitive and volitional capacities. Once again, the shadow of scientific reductionism is implied in this view of the self more as object than as both subject and object.

THE INFLUENCE OF EXISTENTIAL PHILOSOPHY ON PSYCHOTHERAPY

As Frankl, Yalom and others have pointed out, the nature of neurosis and, thus, of appropriate therapeutic intervention has changed since the days of Freud. A large number of complaints for which patients now seek help derive from a lack of meaning in life, and the search for such meaning is what brings such patients to treatment. Since existential philosophy maintains that the only true absolute is that there are no absolutes, this poses a fundamental question: "How does a person who needs meaning find meaning in a universe that has none?"

For centuries, of course, this answer has been found in the positing of a God-centered universe in which man's purpose was to relate to and, if possible, emulate that God. Since this is patently impossible on an individual basis, most philosophers and theologians have arrived at the point of view, exemplified by the work of Teilhard de Chardin (1955), that each individual, by recognizing and joining in this cosmic union, is provided with a personal sense of meaning. At the same time, Kant's questioning of the existence of any fixed, objective reality calls such a view into question. Indeed, Camus and Sartre regard the tension between human aspiration and world indifference as the absurdity of "la condition humaine." Satir refers to this as "the cosmic joke," but maintains that the development of a sense of self-worth enables one to tolerate the irony and to find meaning in the principle of the seed and organic growth.

Viktor Frankl

Frankl (1985) clearly acknowledges his existential debt, coining the word logotherapy ("logos," word or meaning) to indicate his central concern with the problem of meaning. He takes issue with Freud's belief in the homeostatic principle, believing it to be basically reductionist and, therefore, limited in explaining many aspects of human life. Frankl (1963) claims that what man desires "is not a tensionless state, but, rather, a striving and struggling for some goal worthy of him" (p. 166).

Frankl ventures a negative response to the idea of self-actualization, stating that it is an effect and not an object of intention. He believes that "la condition humaine"—the insurmountable finitude of being human—is overcome only when man is able to accept his finiteness. "The whole phenomenon of human existence . . . is inevitable and cannot be circumscribed except by the sentence 'I am'" (Frankl, p. 62). Rather than self-actualization, he would favor self-transcendence as the essence of existence.

He believes that the psychotherapist is not a teacher or preacher, or even a painter. "It is never up to the therapist to convey to the patient a picture of the world as the therapist sees it; but, rather, the therapist should enable the patient to see the world as it is" (ibid., p. 66). In this sense, he endorses the therapeutic use of "maieutic" dialogue in the Socratic sense.

R.D. Laing

Freely acknowledging his roots in existentialism, R.D. Laing (1965, 1969) has written extensively on the role of the self in understanding psychosis. Postulating a "real" self and a "false" self, he believes that the failure to successfully identify each and to distinguish between them is characteristic of patients with schizophrenia. While these distinctions resemble Buber's "being" and "seeming" and Sartre's "real" and "imaginary" selves, Laing speaks further of the "embodied" and the "unembodied" self. In the latter, "the body is felt—more as one object among other objects than as the core of (one's) own being." This deprives "the unembodied self from direct participation in any aspect of the life of the world" (Laing, 1965, p. 69). Thus, "the individual's actions are not felt as expressions of his self" (ibid., p. 74).

Like Buber, Laing is deeply concerned with the act of confirmation, stating "the sense of identity requires the existence of another by whom one is known; and a conjunction of this other person's recognition of one's self with self-recognition" (ibid., p. 139). Lack of confirmation, or disconfirmation, from both self and others is seen as leading to the "chaotic non-entity" of the schizophrenic, where there is total loss of relatedness with both self and other.

Laing believes that the task in therapy is to make contact with the true self of the patient through understanding the existential world of the false self. He quotes Jung as saying that the schizophrenic ceases to be schizophrenic when he meets someone by whom he feels understood. This does not mean that the self-being of the other is known or experienced directly, but that the self-being of the other is existentially confirmed. He quotes Buber as saying "the wish of every man (is) to be confirmed as what he is, even as what he can become." Such confirmation must come from the "true" self of the therapist if it is to truly confirm the "true" self of the patient. True confirmation, however, does not mean agreeing with the patient's illusions or delusions—a destructive act of collusion on the part of the therapist—but, rather, affirming both his being and becoming, and confirming the validity of his unique experience. With Buber, he believes that "an empty claim for confirmation, without devotion for being or becoming, again and again mars the truth of life between man and man." He agrees with Heidegger (1949) that the truth of science, which consists of correspondence between what goes on "in intellectu" and what goes on "in re"—between the structure in the mind and that in the world—is not the same truth as described by the pre-Socratics, where truth is "that which is without secrecy, that discloses itself without a veil" (Laing, 1969, p. 129). Indeed, it may well be the experience of this latter truth through the authentic use of the self which brings validity to the former.

Carl Rogers

To underscore his perception of the person seeking help as basically self-responsible and self-directing, in the late 1930s, Carl Rogers (1951, 1961a, 1961b, 1986) began to use the word "client" rather than "patient." Characteristics of "client-centered psychotherapy," as it came to be known, included a stress on the self-actualizing quality of the person, a concern with the process rather than the structure of personality change, a view of psychotherapy as but one specialized example of constructive interpersonal relationships, a focus on the inner phenomenological world of the client, and an emphasis on the immediacy of the therapist's presence and attitudes, rather than on skills or techniques as key elements in the process of therapy. Based on his observations, Rogers specified three basic attitudes or conditions he believes are important for the success of therapy: the therapist's authenticity, genuineness and congruence, his complete acceptance and "unconditional positive regard" for the client, and his sensitive and empathetic understanding.

Thus, for Rogers, the effective therapist should strive to be totally and authentically himself—without pretense—directly available to the client in a personal sense. In addition, through an attitude of "unconditional positive regard," he should endeavor to create a non-threatening context for therapy, in which it is possible for the client to explore and experience his most deeply hidden feelings. Finally, Rogers believes that therapy is facilitated when the therapist is sensitive on a moment-to-moment basis to the universe of the client and is able to sense and understand the latter's unique and personal learnings as if they were his own. Some of his current ideas on the use of the self in therapy are contained in another chapter in this book.

One of Rogers' major contributions, however, has been his insistence on research to back up his observations. Believing that the phenomenon of therapy can and should be subjected to rigorous investigation, he pioneered in the use of audio and film recordings of actual therapeutic interviews. Results of these investigations have provided data confirming the hypothesis that the attitudes and behavior of the therapist are important elements in therapeutic movement and change.

Existential Psychotherapy

It is not surprising that many serious philosophers have disavowed identification as existentialists, because, as Tillich (1961) has pointed out, "There is not, and cannot be, an existentialist system of philosophy" (p. 9). " Existentialism is an element within a larger frame of essentialism." Like most other philosophical concepts, each view achieves definition only in terms of its opposite, and neither can be totally accepted without inviting rebuttal from the other. Thus, the apparent triumph of existentialism in the 20th century must be seen in an historical perspective which considers and balances the opposing views of idealistic or naturalistic essentialism.

Such a philosophical distinction has tremendous implications for psychotherapy. While it is man's problems which bring him into therapy, it is important to distinguish between those related to his daily life and relationships and those arising from his basic existential anxiety. The former are the appropriate concern and within the usual competence of most therapies and therapists, but psychotherapy cannot cure the existential anxiety which arises from the awful awareness of man's own finitude—"la condition humaine"—although, it can attempt to give meaning to life. It does this in a uniquely human way—through offering the seeker of help the self of the therapist as a significant symbol of faith and hope in the former's effort to bridge the finite and infinite. Buber's "I-Thou" relationship offers precisely this uniquely human act and experience of confirmation.

The existentially-oriented psychotherapist, then, does not manifest a particular technique or theory, nor are the valuable contributions of other psychological theories denied. Rather, a selective approach is used, the central process of therapy being perceived as that of experiencing the full awareness of one's being. Experiential awareness takes precedence over cognitive awareness, the "here and now" is emphasized rather than the past life of the patient, and therapy is regarded as a creative, evolving process of self-discovery. In relating to the patient, the therapist tries to establish a personal bond of trust and meaningful collaboration, based on a genuine belief in his own potentialities and those of the patient. While remaining observing and objective, he attempts to enter the world of his patient, wrestling with the frustrations and limitations of the therapeutic situation, trying to be fully present and subjectively real (Polanyi, 1966). So far as possible, he attempts to manifest Martin Buber's "I-Thou" relationship of mutuality, seeking to liberate the individual to seek and achieve his own optimal development. In short, the existential therapist functions as a fully-available person in a meaningful encounter with another. As Tillich (1961) holds, "a person becomes a person in the encounter with other persons, and in no other way. . . . This interdependence of man and man in the process of becoming human is a judgment against a psychotherapeutic method in which the patient is a mere object for the analyst as subject" (p. 15).

It appears, then, that for the existentially-oriented psychotherapist, the use of self is an essential element in therapy, whether it be with individuals, groups or families. Support for this position has come from the growing influence of general systems theory in psychiatry, which posits that the therapist must be viewed as an integral part of the therapeutic system and as having major effect on the system of the patient. What often is overlooked is that this is a two-way street. In general, this aspect is easier to observe and accept in group and family therapy, where the very number and complexity of the transactions involved make cognitive or technical control of the situation difficult at best. In such situations, it may be more effective for the therapist to "go with the flow"—Buber's musical or floating relationship—and to focus on the metamessages of the system and of his own internal state of being.

This is not a passive process. An attitude of alert, active, attentiveness is required to maintain the essential qualities of contact and receptivity. Nor does this imply control over the situation or over the patient through authority or technique. Rather, the central core of being within the therapist—his very sense of self—serves to communicate and maintain a centering and stabilizing force or power in the process. While such an approach would appear to abdicate the traditional role of the therapist and encourage chaos to take over, this very act of relinquishment of control is precisely what many patients seem to require in order to rediscover and reassert their own sense of control over their lives. At the same time, this act loses its authenticity if used solely as a technique. It is an intensely real and personal act—that of letting go—putting one's belief in one's self and in the self of the other on the line—exposing one's true and deepest self, in a sense, going naked into the encounter—allowing oneself to become truly vulnerable. This "centered act of the centered self" is truly the source of the creative and life-giving act of self-discovery and transformation (Tillich, 1961). Paradoxically, such a use of self implies a deliberate "non-use" or suspension of self in its usual sense.

Achieving and maintaining such an attitude is never easy, and is impossible for some therapists, whose personal needs or belief systems require them to be "in charge." Nor is it the province of any one school or theory. Great therapists of all persuasions have always manifested the essential elements of this quality. Nor does it mean that knowledge, skill and experience are not important. The plethora of self-appointed helpers and "gurus" and the unfortunate results of many pseudotherapies and encounter groups led by non-professionals attest otherwise.

Can such an attitude be learned or acquired? Despite the existence of "natural" healers and therapists, the answer is strongly in the affirmative. Ideally, the training analysis was intended to accomplish this. Unfortunately, it also modeled the traditional authoritarian, or subject-object relationship, and usually ignored significant dimensions of the self of the analyst in training (as well as of the training analyst!). This resulted in perpetuating, for too long, a focus on technique and theory which often obscured the deeply personal relationship involved. Such lessons need to be learned experientially through intense encounter with others, who are able to share openly in their own continuing search. While the ultimate learning experience is always deeply personal, it almost always occurs in relation to another person. Buber has said that the greatest thing one human being can do for another is to confirm the deepest thing within him. It is this act of confirmation which is ultimately implied in the use of self in therapy.

NOTES

1. Arieti, S. (1967). The Intrapsychic Self. New York: Basic Books.
2. Aristotle (1957). On the Soul, (Trans. by Hett, W.S.). Cambridge: Harvard Univ. Press.
3. Buber, M. (1923). Ich und Du. Leipzig: Insel-Verlag
4. Buber, M. (1955). *Between Man and Man*, (Trans. by Smith, R.G.). Boston: Beacon Press.
5. Buber, M. (1965). *The Knowledge of Man: A Philosophy of the Interhuman.* New York: Harper & Row.
6. Buber, M. (1970). *I and Thou.* New York: Charles Scribners.
7. de Chardin, T. (1955). *The Phenomenon of Man.* New York: Harper.
8. Erikson, E.H. (1950). *Childhood and Society.* New York: Norton.
9. Erikson, E.H. (1959). *Identity and the Life Cycle.* New York: Int'l. Univ. Press.
10. Fink, D.L. (1979). Holistic Health: The Evolution of Western Medicine, pp. 1-12. In *A Humanistic Perspective on Holistic Health Values,* publ. by Western Colorado Health Systems Agency.
11. Frankl, V.E. (1963). Man's Search for Meaning: An Introduction to Logotherapy. New York: Pocket Books.
12. Frankl, V.E. (1985). *Psychotherapy and Existentialism.* New York: Washington Square Press.
13. Freud, S. (1934). The Unconscious. In *Collected Papers,* Vol. 4. London: Hogarth.
14. Friedman, M. (1965). Introductory Essay. In Buber, M., *The Knowledge of Man.* New York: Harper & Row.
15. Greenacre, P. (1958). Early Physical Determinants in the Development of a Sense of Identity. *JAPA* 6:612-627.
16. Heidegger, M. (1962). *Being and Time.* New York: Harper & Row.
17. Hollender, M. & Szasz, T.S. (1956).' A Contribution to the Philosophy of Medicine. *Arch. Int. Med.,* 97:585-592.
18. Horney, K. (1939). *New Ways in Psychoanalysis.* New York: Norton.
19. Horney, K. (1950). *Neurosis and Human Growth.* New York: Norton.
20. Husserl, E. (1965). *Phenomenology and the Crisis of Philosophy.* New York: Harper & Row.
21. Jung, C.G. (1971). *Psychological Types.* Princeton: Bollingen Series 20.
22. Kernberg, O. Contemporary Controversies Regarding the Concept of the Self. Unpublished paper, quoted in Cooper, A.M., Chap. 15, in *Handbook of Psychiatry,* 2nd Ed., Arieti, S. (Ed.) 1974, New York: Basic Books.
23. Kierkegaard, S. (1959). *Either/Or,* 2 vols. New York: Doubleday, Anchor.
24. Kohut, H. (1971). *The Analysis of the Self.* New York: Int'l. Univ. Press.
25. Kohut, H. (1985). *Self Psychology and the Humanities.* Strozier, C.B., (Ed.). New York: W.W. Norton.
26. Laing, R.D. (1965). *The Divided Self.* Baltimore: Penguin Books.
27. Laing, R.D. (1969). *Self and Others.* New York: Penguin Books.
28. Maslow, A. (1962). *Toward a Psychology of Being.* New York: Van Nostrand.
29. Mead, G.H. (1934). *Mind, Self and Society.* Chicago: Univ. Chicago Press.
30. Polanyi, M. (1966). *The Tacit Dimension.* New York: Doubleday.
31. Roccatagliata, G. (1986). *A History of Ancient Psychiatry.* New York: Greenwood.
32. Rogers, G. (1951). *Client-Centered Therapy.* Boston: Houghton-Mifflin.
33. Rogers, C. (1961a). The Process Equation of Psychotherapy. *Am. J. Psychotherapy* 14: 27-45.
34. Rogers, G. (1961b). *On Becoming a Person.* Boston: Houghton-Mifflin.
35. Rogers, C. (1961c). Two Divergent Trends. In *Existential Psychology,* Rollo May, (Ed.). New York: Random House, Inc.
36. Rogers, C. (1986). (In press. This volume.)
37. Sartre, J.P. (1956). *Being and Nothingness* (Trans. by Barnes, H.). New York: Philosophical Library.
38. Sartre, J.P. (1950). *Psychology of Imagination.* London: Rider.
39. Spiegel, L. (1959). The Self, The Sense of Self and Perception. Psa. Stc 14.
40. Standal, S. & Corsini, R., Eds. (1959). *Critical Incidents in Psychotherapy.* Englewood Cliffs, NJ: Prentice Hall.

41. Strupp, H.H. (1958). The Psychotherapist's Contribution to the Treatment Process. *Behav. Sci.* 3:34-67.

42. Strupp, H.H. (1963). The Outcome Problem in Psychotherapy Revisited. *Psychotherapy* 1:1-13.

43. Strupp, H.H. (1973). Specific vs. Non-Specific Factors in Psychotherapy and the Problem of Control. In Strupp, H.H., (Ed.), *Psychotherapy: Clinical, Research and Theoretical Issues.* New York: Jason Aronson, pp. 103-121.

44. Sullivan, H.S. (1953). *The Interpersonal Theory of Psychiatry.* New York: Norton.

45. Tillich, P. (1952). *The Courage to Be.* New Haven: Yale Press.

46. Tillich, P. (1961). Existentialism and Psychotherapy. *Rev. Existent, Psychol. and Psychiat.* 1:8-16.

47. Truax, C.B., Wargo, D., Frank, J., Imber, S., Battle, C., Hoehn-Saric, R., Nash, E., & Stone, A. (1966a). The Therapist's Contribution to Accurate Empathy, Non-Possessive Warmth, and Genuineness in Psychotherapy. *J. Clin. Psychol.* 22:331-334.

48. Truax, C.B., Wargo, D., Frank, J., Imber, S., Battle, C., Hoehn-Saric, R., Nash, E., & Stone, A. (1966b). Therapist Empathy, Genuineness and Warmth, and Patient Therapeutic Outcome. *J. Consult. Psychol.* 30:395-401.

49. Wolpe, J. (1961). The Prognosis in Unpsychoanalyzed Recovery from Neurosis. *Am. J. Psychiat.* 118:35.

50. Yalom, I. (1980). *Existential Psychotherapy.* New York: Basic Books, Inc.

Interview with Carl Rogers
On the Use of the Self in Therapy

Michele Baldwin

Carl Rogers on account of his leading role in the field of humanistic psychology, was the first psychotherapist whom we asked to be a contributor to this special issue. He felt that his busy schedule did not allow him to contribute a paper at this time. Because of his interest in this area, however, he suggested as an alternative to be interviewed on this topic. These words were spoken during a relaxed morning in his living room.

Over time, I think that I have become more aware of the fact that in therapy I do use myself. I recognize that when I am intensely focused on a client, just my presence seems to be healing and I think this is probably true of any good therapist. I recall once I was working with a schizophrenic man in Wisconsin whom I had dealt with over a period of a year or two and there were many long pauses. The crucial turning point was when he had given up, did not care whether he lived or died, and was going to run away from the institution. And I said; "I realize that you don't care about yourself, but I want you to know that I care about you, and I care what happens to you." He broke into sobs for 10 or 15 minutes. That was the turning point of the therapy. I had responded to his feelings and accepted them but it was when I came to him as a person and expressed my feelings for him, that it really got to him. That interested me, because I am inclined to think that in my writing perhaps I have stressed too much the three basic conditions (congruence, unconditional positive regard and empathic understanding). Perhaps it is something around the edges of those conditions that is really the most important element of therapy—when my self is very clearly, obviously present.

When I am working, I know that there is a lot of active energy flowing from me to the client, and I am now aware that it probably was present to some degree from the first. I remember a client whose case I have written up, who said towards the end of therapy: "I don't know a thing about you, and, yet, I have never known any one so well," I think that is an important element, that even though a client did not know my age or my family or other details of my life, I became well known to her as a person.

In using myself, I include my intuition and the essence of myself, whatever that is. It is something very subtle, because myself as a person has a lot of specific characteristics that do not enter in as much as just the essential elements of myself. I also include my caring, and my ability to really listen acceptantly. I used to think that was easy. It has taken me a long time to realize that for me, for most people, this is extremely hard. To listen acceptantly, no matter what is being voiced, is a rare thing and is something I try to do.

When I am with a client, I like to be aware of my feelings, and if there are feelings which run contrary to the conditions of therapy and occur persistently, then I am sure I want to express them. But there are also other feelings. For instance, sometimes, with a woman client, I feel: "this woman is sexually attractive, I feel attracted to her." I would not express that unless it comes up as an issue in therapy. But, if I felt annoyed by the fact that she was always complaining, let us say, and I kept feeling annoyed, then, I would express it.

The important thing is to be aware of one's feeling and then you can decide whether it needs to be expressed or is appropriate to express. Sometimes, it is amusing. I know in one demonstration interview, I suddenly was aware of something about the recording. I believe they had not turned on the recorder or something like that. It was just a flash and then I was back with the client. In discussing it afterwards, I said: "there was one moment when I really was not with you." And he replied: "Yes, I knew that." It is very evident when there is a break in a relationship like that. I did not express that concern because it seemed irrelevant and yet, it was relevant. It would have been better had I said: "For a moment there, I was thinking about the machine, and now I am back with you."

I think that the therapist has a right to his or her own life. One of the worst things is for a therapist to permit the client to take over, or to be a governing influence in the therapist's life. It happened to me once, and was nearly disastrous. It was with a schizophrenic client of whom I got tired, I guess. I had done some good work with her—and sometimes not—and she sort of clung to me, which I resented, but did not express. Gradually she came to know me well enough to know just how to press my buttons and she kept me very upset. In fact, I began to feel that she knew me better than I knew myself, and that obviously is non-therapeutic and disastrous to the therapist. It helped me to realize that one of the first requirements for being a therapist is that there be a live therapist. I think it is important to realize that one has a need and a right to preserve and protect oneself. A therapist has a right to give, but not to get worn out trying to be giving. I think different therapists have different kinds of boundaries: Some can give a great deal and really not harm themselves, and others find it difficult to do that.

A number of years ago, I would have said that the therapist should not be a model to the client—that the client should develop his or her own

[handwritten: therapist as model]

models, and I still feel that to some degree. But, in one respect, the therapist is a model. By listening acceptantly to every aspect of the client's experience, the therapist is modeling the notion of listening to oneself. And,
by being accepting and non-judgmental of the feelings within the client,
the therapist is modelling a non-judgmental self acceptance in the client.
By being real and congruent and genuine, the therapist is modelling that
kind of behavior for the client. In these ways, the therapist does serve as a
useful model.

The way I am perceived by the client also makes a difference, but not
in the therapeutic process. If I am seen as a father figure, for example,
then that makes a difference in the therapy; it makes a difference in the
client's feelings. But, since the whole purpose of therapy, as I see it, is to
hear and accept and recognize the feelings that the client is having, it does
not make much fundamental difference whether the client sees me as a
young person or a lover, or as a father figure, as long as the client is able
to express some of those feelings. The process is the same regardless of
which feelings are being experienced.

This is why I differ so fundamentally with the psychoanalysts on this
business of transference. I think it is quite natural that a client might feel
positive feelings towards the therapist. There is no reason to make a big
deal out of it. It can be handled in the same way as the fact that the client
might be afraid of the therapist, or of his or her father. Any feelings are
grist for the mill as far as therapy is concerned, providing the client can
express them and providing the therapist is able to listen acceptantly. I
think the whole concept of transference got started because the therapist
got scared when the client began to feel strong positive or negative feelings towards the therapist.

The whole process of therapy is a process of self-exploration, of getting acquainted with one's own feelings and coming to accept them as a
part of the self. So, whether the feelings are in regard to the parents, or in
regard to the therapist, or in regard to some situation, it really makes no
difference. The client is getting better acquainted with and becoming
more accepting of his or herself and that can be true with regard to the
transference feelings. When the client realizes: "Yes, I do love him very
much," or whatever, and accepts those as a real part of self, the process
of therapy advances.

I think that therapy is most effective when the therapist's goals are
limited to the process of therapy and not the outcome. I think that if the
therapist feels "I want to be as present to this person as possible. I want to
really listen to what is going on. I want to be real in this relationship,"
then these are suitable goals for the therapist. If the therapist is feeling, "I
want this person to get over this neurotic behavior, I want this person to
change in such and such a way," I think that stands in the way of good
therapy. The goal has to be within myself, with the way I am. Once thera-

py is under way, another goal of the therapist's is to question: "Am I really with this person in this moment? Not where they were a little while ago, or where are they going to be, but am I really with this client in this moment." This is the most important thing.

Another important element is the maturity of the therapist. I recall that in Chicago, a graduate student did some research that seemed to indicate that the more psychologically mature the therapist, the more effective the therapy was likely to be. It was not a definitive research, but I suspect that there is a lot of truth in it. Not only experience in living, but what one has done with that experience in living makes a difference in therapy. It ties in with another feeling I have—that perhaps I am good at helping people to recognize their own capacities, because I have come to value and represent the notion of self-empowerment. However, somebody else may be good at helping them in another way, because they have achieved maturity in another realm. What I am saying is that different therapists have different characteristics of their mature personality and probably these different elements help clients move in those directions.

The mature person is always open to all of the evidence coming in, and that means open to continuing change. Often people ask me: "How have you changed over the years?" And I can see from the way they phrase their question that they are asking "What have I rejected, what have I thrown away." Well, I haven't rejected much of anything, but I have been astonished at the fact that those ideas which started in individual therapy could have such very wide implications and applications.

My career as a therapist has gone through a number of phases. One of the earliest and most important was when I gave up on a mother and her son. My staff was handling the boy and I was dealing with the mother, trying to get across to her the fact that her problem was her rejection of the boy. We went through a number of interviews and I had learned to be quite attentive and gentle. I had been trying to get this point of view across but I was not succeeding, so I said, "I think we both have tried, but this is not working, so we might as well call it quits. Do you agree?" She indicated that she thought so, too. She said "goodbye" and walked to the door. Then she turned and said: "Do you ever take adults for counselling here?" I said "yes," and with that she came back and began to pour out her story of problems with her husband, which was so different from the nice case history I had been taking that I could hardly recognize it. I did not know quite what to do with it, and I look back at this as being the first real therapy case that I ever handled. She kept in touch with me for a long time. The problems with the boy cleared up. I felt is was successful therapy, but did not quite know how it came about.

Later, another change occurred. I had been impressed by Rankian thinking. We had him in for a two day workshop and I liked it. So, I decided to hire a social worker who was a product of the Philadelphia

School of Social Work, Elizabeth Davis. It was from her that I first got the idea of responding to feelings, of respecting feelings—whether she used that terminology or not I am not sure. I don't think she learned very much from me, but I learned a lot from her.

Then, another steppingstone. I had long been interested in recording interviews, but it was very difficult to do in those days. The equipment required that somebody be in another room, recording three minutes on the face of a record and then brushing off the shavings of glass, since we could not get metal during the war. Then, they had to turn the record over and continue. Anyway, it was really difficult. But, when we began to analyze these interviews—and we gradually got better equipment—it was astounding what we learned from these microscopic examinations of the interviews. One could clearly see where an interview had been going along smoothly—the process flowing—and then one response on the part of the counselor just switched things off for a while, or perhaps for the whole interview. We also began to see that some of the people in my practicum came to be called "blitz" therapists, because they would seem to have a couple of very good interviews with their clients, and then the client never came back. It was not until we examined the recordings that we realized that the therapist had been too good, had gone too far, revealed too much of the client's inner-self to them and scared the hell out of them. Another important development in my career was the writing of a very rigorous theory of the client-centered approach. I was very excited that what had gradually been developing quite experientially, could be put into tight cognitive terms which could be tested. This gave me a great deal of confidence, and a great deal of satisfaction. Another change in my career occurred when I moved out to California. Having had the opportunity to realize the power of relatively brief intensive group experiences, I directed my energy to the development of intensive encounter groups. I also developed the applications of my theories to education, and then to large groups.

Finally, early in life I acquired a strong belief in a democratic point of view, and that belief has impacted my therapy. I became convinced that the final authority lies with the individual and that there is no real external authority that can be depended upon. It comes down to one's internal choice, made with all the evidence that one can get and the best possible way that one can cope.

I have always been able to rely on the fact that if I can get through the shell, if I can get through to the person there will be a positive and constructive inner core. That is why I hold a different point of view from Rollo May. He seems to feel that there is a lot of essential evil in the individual, but I have never been able to pin him down as to whether it is genetic or not. I feel that if people were evil, I would be shocked or horrified at what I found if I was able to get through to the core of that person.

I have never had that experience—just the opposite. If I can get through to
a person, even those whose behavior has a lot of destructive elements, I
believe he or she would want to do the right thing. So I do not believe that
people are genetically evil. Something must have happened after birth to
warp them. It has often been said that I could not work with psychopaths,
because they have no social conscience. Well, my feeling is: yes, it would
be difficult and I don't think they would come easily into one-to-one psychotherapy. But if they could be part of a group for a long period of time,
then I think they could probably be gotten to.

Recently my views have broadened into a new area about which I
would like to comment. A friend, who is a minister, always kids me about
the fact that I am one of the most spiritual people he knows, but I won't
admit it. Another time, a group of young priests were trying to pin me to
the wall, saying that I must be religious. I finally said to them and it is
something I still stand by—"I am too religious to be religious," and that
has quite a lot of meaning for me. I have my own definition of spirituality.
I would put it that the best of therapy sometimes leads to a dimension that
is spiritual, rather than saying that the spiritual is having an impact on
therapy. But it depends on your definition of spiritual. There are certainly
times in therapy and in the experience I have had with groups where I feel
that there is something going on that is larger than what is evident. I have
described this in various ways. Sometimes I feel much as the physicists,
who do not really split atoms; they simply align themselves up in accordance with the natural way in which the atoms split themselves. In the
same way, I feel that sometimes in interpersonal relationships power and
energy get released which transcends what we thought was involved.

As I recently said, I find that when I am the closest to my inner, intuitive self—when perhaps I am somehow in touch with the unknown in
me—when perhaps I am in a slightly altered state of consciousness in the
relationship, then, whatever I do seems to be full of healing. Then simply
my presence is releasing and helpful. At those moments, it seems that my
inner spirit has reached out and touched the inner spirit of the other. Our
relationship transcends itself, and has become part of something larger.
Profound growth and healing and energy are present.

To be a fully authentic therapist, I think that you have to feel entirely
secure as a person. This allows you to let go of yourself, knowing confi-
dently that you can come back. Especially when you work with a group,
you have to surrender yourself to a process of which you are a part and
admit you can't have a complete understanding. And then when you get to
dealing with a group of 500 or 600, you surrender any hope of understanding what is going on and, yet, by surrendering yourself to the process, certain things happen.

The therapist needs to recognize very clearly the fact that he or she is
an imperfect person with flaws which make him vulnerable. I think it is

only as the therapist views himself as imperfect and flawed that he can see himself as helping another person. Some people who call themselves therapists are not healers, because they are too busy defending themselves.

The self I use in therapy does not include all my personal characteristics. Many people are not aware that I am a tease and that I can be very tenacious and tough, almost obstinate. I have often said that those who think I am always gentle should get into a fight with me, because they would find out quite differently. I guess that all of us have many different facets, which come into play in different situations. I am just as real when I am understanding and accepting, as when I am being tough. To me being congruent means that I am aware of and willing to represent the feelings I have at the moment. It is being real and authentic in the moment.

I am frequently asked what kind of training is necessary to become a person-centered therapist. I know some very good person-centered therapists who have had no training at all! I think that one could go to small remote villages and find out who people turn to for help, what are the characteristics of these people they turn to? I think to be a good person-centered therapist, one needs to experience a person-centered approach either in an intensive group for some period of time, or in individual therapy, or whatever. I don't, however, believe in requiring such an experience. I feel that the opportunity should be available, but not required.

Then, in addition to that, I think that breadth of learning is perhaps the most important. I'd rather have someone who read widely and deeply in literature or in physics, than to have someone who has always majored in psychology in order to become a therapist. I think that breadth of learning along with breadth of life experience are essential to becoming a good therapist. Another thing: the importance of recording interviews cannot be overestimated. Videotaping is even better, although I have not had much experience with that. But, to have the opportunity to listen to what went on, be it right after the interview or one year later, to try to understand the process of what went on, should be a tremendous learning experience. I think that one should let the beginning therapist do what ever he wants in therapy, provided that he records the sessions and listens to them afterwards, so that he can see the effects on the process. I think that the careful review of recorded interviews is essential.

recorded interviews are essential for the beginning therapist

I think that my present viewpoints are difficult to admit in academic circles. In the past, I could be understood at a purely cognitive level. However, as I became clearer as to what I was doing, academicians had to allow room for experiential learning, which is quite threatening, because, then, the instructor might have to become a learner, which is not popular in such circles. I think it is much easier to accept me as someone who had some ideas in the 40s that can be described, than try to understand what has been happening since. I know very few people in major universities who have any real or deep understanding of my work. In some of the external degree institutions, yes, and outside of institutions there are a number of such people. It is interesting that the degree of understanding does not depend on the degree of contact with me. When people are philosophically ready for that part of me, they can pick it up entirely from reading. If they are not philosophically ready, they can do an awful lot of reading and still not get the point. Basically, it is a way of being, and universities are not interested in ways of being. They are more interested in ideas and ways of thinking.

People have asked me what effect I think my work has had on other professions. I think that my most important impact has been on education. I don't feel that I have had much influence on medicine or psychiatry or even on psychology. I have had much more influence in counseling, but not on the main stream of psychology. I think I have had some impact on nursing. Nurses don't need to defend themselves against change and new ideas. I am also intrigued with the thought that the idea of leaving a human being free to follow his own choices is gradually extending into business.

Finally, I have been interested to see an evolution in the practice of medicine, where the idea of empowering the patient has brought medicine "back" to the idea that patients can heal themselves. I am also pleased to see the development of personal responsibility in health. One of the most important things is that we have opened up psychotherapy and substituted the growth model for the medical model.

The Differing Self:
Women as Psychotherapists

Helen V. Collier

ABSTRACT. Family therapy needs to consider the impact of the large numbers of women bringing "self" to the therapeutic process as both therapists and family members. The cautious and disciplined use of the self is an inevitable and invaluable aid to the therapist. It is inevitable because of biological, sociological, political, and experiential differences in the development of females and males. It is invaluable because it enables the flexibility of therapeutic response which clients deserve, particularly in the matter of "the different voice" with which women speak.

"The failure to see the different reality of women's lives and to hear the differences in their voices stems in part from the assumption that there is a single mode of social experience and interpretation. By positing instead two different modes, we arrive at a more complex rendition of human experience . . . " (Carol Gilligan, 1982, p. 173).

Accounts of the "what I do in therapy" variety usually come to grief on the twin reefs of egoism and tedium, but as a practitioner my contribution to this collection of writings about the use of self in psychotherapy has to be personal rather than scholastic. What follows, therefore, seeks to avoid those perilous twin reefs by summarizing what I think happens when any of us engage in psychotherapy. My own special aid to navigation is what happens differently when the therapist is a female.

Throughout my professional career, there has always been argument about whether a therapist should reveal self and personal values in the psychotherapeutic relationship or stay aloof and "objective," relying on scientifically replicable techniques to accomplish the intervention and achieve the clients' goals. I've seen all the "schools" of therapy at work, and I've watched several therapists switch from one side of the debate to the other. The need to remain "objective" and the usefulness of replica-

Helen V. Collier, Ed.D., is a Counseling Psychologist and Marriage and Family Counselor. After some twenty years as a therapist, she now specializes in working with family systems, small work units, and the management of large organizations both private and public.

She is the author of *Counseling Women: A Guide for Therapists* (1982), *Freeing Ourselves* (1981), and numerous articles. She is a member of the American Psychological Association, the Women's Equity Action League, and the International Human Learning Resources Network. Address reprint requests to Dr. Collier at P.O. Box 2809, Reno, NV 89505.

ble techniques have always been an invaluable sheet-anchor in my practice. But I have never made them my chief goal, and, for reasons stem-
ming from my educational background, the general debate has amused
more often than it has engaged me.

Educated young in religion and literature, and later in the philosophy of
science, I seem always to have believed—like those disciplines—that absolute objectivity does not exist in human relationships even if the search
for it should often be their goal. Once my academic education in Psychology Departments was complete, it came as a relief to train with Erving
and Miriam Polster, for they were very clear about a premise I was happy
to accept: that technique and technology are not the center of the therapeutic process but should be present only to enrich the effect of the psychotherapist in the process by which our clients (whether individuals,
couples, families, or groups) heal and grow.

No matter what "technique" I use in my own practice (and I use
many), central to everything is my personal presence in the process and
my awareness of who I am and how I use that presence. But the reef of
egoism immediately looms dead ahead! To dominate clients with my own
self is to be a rotten therapist. The therapist's ego is a bore and a distrac-
tion. It is the clients' success, not my own, that I must seek. If I become
central or dominant, then I guarantee failure in the goal of facilitating
their process and experience. Here, then, is the dilemma of the personal
approach and the danger of reliance on the use of self.

Far from sinking us, however, that reef makes us navigate better. The
awareness of the dilemma of self is the most valuable technique a therapist can have. I find that as long as I am fully conscious of myself as well
as my clients during the therapeutic process, I am able to make clear
choices as to the role I will play with these individuals in this particular
situation. Those roles vary greatly: consultant, catalyst, resource-
provider, reactor, observer, problem-solver, sharing human, sometimes
even just a shoulder to cry on. From minute to minute, through awareness
and accompanying discomfort, I often receive cues to change roles.

The steady awareness I seek during a psychotherapeutic session is
something I can only call "healthy energy." The normal human experience is total presence in the world, constant interaction with a multitude
of stimuli in the environment and the physiological self, steady exchange
of energy in a great variety of ways. The therapist, I believe, should always attempt to enhance that normal experience in herself or himself during therapy. How? By staying aware that during therapy the whole composite of her or his experiences (past, present, future) is at work, that all
the hopes and failures, all the expertise and ignorance, all the perceptions
of self both in the therapeutic process and in the world, all the understanding of the intricacy of being alive is functioning in the here and now between this therapist and this family, couple, or individual client. The dif-

ference between therapist and non-therapist, I believe, is the degree of consciousness and responsiveness to the interaction between organism and environment.

Let me look at this belief from the viewpoint of a woman. I recently attended a professional conference in which a question was posed to some thirty psychotherapists, mostly women. The speaker asked why, in a profession where so many practitioners are female, are so small a proportion of the profession's leaders female. Why were so few women major theorists and significant conceptualizers? Where was the voice of the female family therapist in our profession? The question got no good answer, but it stimulated me to explore possibilities. The answer, I believe, lies in what Carol Gilligan has recently and brilliantly named the "different voice" of women.

Gilligan published her work In a Different Voice in 1982, and the book at once found resonances in several professions. For example, "Portia in a Different Voice" (Menkel-Meadow, 1985) explores the significance of lawyering by women for the legal profession and the legal process. Speculations on the meaning of her approach for family therapy are the main substance of this present article.

As have other empirical scholars, Gilligan challenges the theories of Piaget and Kohlberg as based on male standards and models. Studying the psychological and moral development of women over their lifetimes, she finds that "in view of the evidence that women perceive and constitute reality differently from men and that these differences center around experiences of attachment and separation, life transitions that invariably engage these experiences can be expected to involve women in a distinctive way" (p. 171). But it is her subsequent conclusion from this basis that makes her work new and exciting. She suggests that the silencing of the female voice through ignoring women's different personality development has resulted not just in harm to women but in an impoverishment of our ability to understand humanity, not just women. She convincingly proposes that the sex differences in the personality formation of male and female mean that each sex speaks "in a different voice," and that the blending of those voices is the truly human chorus.

The two sexes are trained to experience and express things differently, writes Gilligan. Masculinity is defined through separation, femininity through attachment. Male gender identity is threatened by intimacy, female gender identity by separation. Whereas Vaillant (1977) and Levinson (1978) found separation and attachment to be distinct stages through which people pass, Gilligan finds this to be true only for men, not for women, for whom the two stages are fused. Males tend to have difficulty with relating, females with individuation. The male identity domain holds tight boundaries for the exercise of exclusion, the female identity domain has loose boundaries for the process of interconnection. Males tend to believe that there is one right way to live and their task is to find it. Females tend to believe that there are many right ways to live and their task is find the right one for now. Inevitably, then, when women and men speak, even of the same thing, they speak in different voices.

Let me give you an example of the implications of these ideas for women both as clients and as psychotherapists. From the male viewpoint, women's inability to separate is, by definition, a failure to "develop." From the female viewpoint, however, the fusion of identity and intimacy is not a developmental failure but a way of living fully. This means that a female therapist and a male therapist could, from the start, view the same female client very differently. Similar differences would affect male and female therapists' views of male clients. And these differences would come before or beneath the differences between therapists as individuals. In sum, the "self" of the therapist could inevitably control the nature of the therapy.

Another example is the concept of morality when it comes to the giving of "care," as in the role of the therapist. Gilligan finds that the male concept of morality emphasizes fairness and ties moral development to the understanding of rights and rules. The female concept of moral development, however, centers around the understanding of responsibility in relationships. Now, imagine a client (male or female) whose basic question is, "What is the right thing to do?" Both the male and the female therapist may hear the same words, but the words will mean utterly different things.

I recognize, of course, that one cannot say that all behavior characteristics belong to one gender or the other. Apart from being stupid, that would perpetuate the stereotypes which prevent us from seeing qualities as qualities regardless of their gender context. Worse, it would camouflage the differences between individual women and individual men that are the very source of richness they bring to the therapeutic process. It would be as narrowing as making a diagnosis and then seeing all of an individual's behavior in terms of that diagnosis only.

On the other hand, empirical research (Maccoby & Jacklin, 1974; Williams, 1982; Gilligan, 1982) and studies of the social process (Horney, 1973; Dweck, 1976; Pleck, 1976; Miller, 1976; Bernard, 1981; Collier, 1982) show that certain values, attitudes, and behavior are related to gender. Differences between the genders exist. If they exist, they have some impact on the self we bring to the therapeutic process and on the experience of that therapeutic process.

Nor am I claiming the female therapist's way to be better than the male therapist's way, since "better" can only be defined in terms of appropriateness to the needs of the clients. I do claim, however, that the female therapist by virtue of her own conditioning is more likely to hear the different voice of the female client. She is also likely to hear more than the male, to be less certain in giving either diagnosis or prescription, and to be less interested in having the client fit a theory or abstract concept.

Rather than exacerbate the fruitless debate as to whether females or males are "better" in some sense, I advocate an expansion of both sexes into the virtues of the other, and a resultant enrichment of our profession's skills. Eventually, I believe, we will have large numbers of therapists who can hear both voices. When life-cycle theorists devote as much attention to females as to males, and when conceptualizers are more equally females and males, then our profession's vision will encompass the experience of both sexes and we will have theories and concepts more fertile than those which presently exist. At that time, the question about women "leaders" in proportion to their professional numbers will no longer be asked.

I would add, however, a note of warning that brings me close to the reef of feminist tedium. Some men listen very well. Many women listen very badly. But for reasons historical, political, economic, and sociological, women learn to listen far more and far better to the voice of men than do men to the voice of women. We have to. It is a matter of the need to function, a matter of power, a matter of survival. The legal and official gains made by women in the last few decades have made barely the slightest change in this area. It is the men more than the women in our profession who need to tune up their hearing aids.

Let me summarize the qualities which, I believe, my female self brings to the therapeutic process.

1. My capacity to use the kind of judgment-perspective typical of women gives me an equal regard for attachment and autonomy.
2. My perspective that there are many ways to deal with a problem, any of which may be acceptable, enables me to help clients choose a "male" or a "female" way appropriate to all needs, not just to biological gender.
3. When a woman in therapy chooses to act on the basis of the caring in a relationship, my recognition that her choices come not just from dependency-needs but from a sense of connectedness to other humans and the need to protect that connectedness enables me to help her face choice with greater consciousness.
4. Aware that every person needs both autonomy and attachment, and with considerable experience in my own life as daughter, lover, wife, mother, worker, and friend at balancing those needs, my flexibility helps clients to decide which quality is appropriate in a particular situation. In therapy this is the real issue more often than is usually admitted.

5. My female training in connecting with others without losing my self makes both me and my clients comfortable with the difficult concept that self-identity and fusion with others are not inimical.

6. My identity as a woman brings an awareness of the female reality that no man can have, the experience that our biology makes us share, our socialization, our sexual development, our work lives, our different sense of the purpose of life.

7. My identity as a woman also gives me the ability to hear and interpret both the female and the male voice, and to act as a translator or trainer.

8. When working with couples separately or with a family, my ability to hear the two voices enables me, first, to clarify their existence and nature. Then I can face the crucial matter of whether to reinforce one voice or the other, to aim at creating harmony between the two, or (on some happy occasions) to encourage a couple or a family to transcend them.

9. Wary of the reef of egoism, however, I much prefer to work with a male co-therapist in couple or family situations. Our joined ability to hear different voices, and our cooperation in tuning them, is often a geometrical increase over either of us working alone or with another therapist of the same sex.

This brief discussion of the different voices and selves brought to the therapeutic process has to end in speculation. Why, for instance, has the female voice gone unheard for so long? What messages does that voice carry which the profession does not want to hear? Or again, are the men in our profession better attuned to the different voices than most men because they are less bound by tradition and better oriented to connections? Or is the reverse true: are they less conventional because they are better attuned? And yet again, can our profession be enriched by paying more attention to the existence of different voices? What really are the lessons we will learn when we hear their symphony? Will they teach that there is a world very different in nature from that bifurcated world we have so far created?

Over my years of private practice, women have come to me mostly with the goal of understanding themselves better and sorting through the complexities which multiple commitments bring to a woman's life. The pattern of men, who have come in steadily increasing numbers, has been different. Those who mostly wanted to understand themselves better used to choose, I believe, a male therapist. For many years, men who came to me were mainly those who felt confusion and frustration in regard to women. Though often starting with the desire to have me "straighten out" their women, they wanted better to understand themselves at most in relationship to women. Then a new breed began to come: men wanting to love and to live with women more effectively, who sensed that they were poor at achieving intimacy. Currently, another group is becoming familiar. These are men who embrace the ethic of caring and attachment and want to do more about it, men who are conscious of the limitations of the male life and want to expand, men unsettled by the generally arid life of work and society instead of just by the troubled home. These are the men who, like women since many years ago, want to understand themselves better and develop a life of balance and fullness. These are the men who understand that what we share as humans is much greater than what separates us as women and men.

I attribute this development not to any change in my own professional reputation but to a change in male attitudes. These men come to a female therapist because they get something from her they cannot get from many male therapists. I think what they seek is the degree and quality of human contact, the feeling of connectedness in a world losing meaning, the lack of hierarchical directiveness, the flexibility that approves a wide variety of choices, and above all the absence of competitive ego. They feel they can benefit from a deeper experience of the female world in the person of their therapist and expand their own male world to the fuller world of being human.

If I'm right, this is pleasant support for saying that the self is crucial to the role of the therapist. The self is not just individual; it is also biological, social, and ethical. It seems transparently clear to me that the most important choice for our clients is not which technique will help them best (though this too is important) but which therapist will offer the widest and most flexible response as an individual to the clients as individuals.

It is just as transparent that the crucial choice for a therapist is to learn to use her or his self with the flexibility and integrity and range that each and every client merits. Sidney Jourard (1971) wrote, "Shall I permit my fellow humans to know me as I truly am or shall I seek instead to remain an enigma and be seen as someone I am not?" For a responsible therapist, the question can have only one answer, but the applications of that answer must be as cautious and painstaking and selfless as possible.

REFERENCES

Bernard, J. (1981). The female world. New York: The Free Press.

Collier, H. (1982). Counseling women: A guide for therapists. New York: The Free Press.

Dweck, C.S. (1976). Children's interpretation of evaluative feedback: The effect of social cues on learned helplessness. *Merril-Palmer Quarterly, 22,* 105-110.

Gilligan, C. (1982). In a different voice. Cambridge, MA: Harvard University Press.

Horney, K. (1973). Feminine psychology. New York: Norton.

Jourard, S. M. (1971). The transparent self. New York: Van Nostrand.

Levinson, D. (1978). The seasons of a man's life. New York: Alfred A. Knopf.

Maccoby, E.E. & Jacklin C.N. (1974). The psychology of sex differences. Stanford: Stanford University Press.

Menkel-Meadow, C. (1985). "Portia in a different voice: Speculations on a women's lawyering process," *Berkeley Women's Law Journal, 1, 39-63.*

Miller, J.B. (1976). *Toward a new psychology of women. Boston: Beacon Press.*

Pleck, J.H. (1976). *The male sex role: Definitions, problems, and sources of change. Journal of Social Issues, 32,* 155-164.

Vaillant, G.E. (1976) Adaptation to life. Boston: Little, Brown.

Williams, J.H. (1982). Psychology of women: Behavior in a biosocial context. New York: W.W. Norton.

The Self in Family Therapy: A Field Guide

David V. Keith

ABSTRACT. The opportunity for continued expansion of one's own personhood is often the attraction underlying the wish to become a professional psychotherapist. Professional training may fail to enhance personhood, but effective therapy depends upon the re-emergence of the therapist's personal self. This paper describes some of the manifestations of the personal self in the work of a family therapist.

Through its several doorways, many enter the psychotherapy profession in an effort to deepen their connection with the Self. Too often, professional training patterns take over and the Self is obscured or put to sleep.

To illustrate, first-year medical students join me in family interviews. I am frequently impressed by their deadly accurate, though unschooled, observations of family dynamics. When they return two years later in their psychiatric rotation, I am again impressed by how distorted the vision of these same students has become. The distorting lens is a theoretical construct (chemical imbalance) or identification with a new world view (science clarifies all experience).

What happens to this Self (whatever It is) with which we seek to deepen our connection? Too often a professional image is erected and the Self is suffocated by education, blinded by theory and burdened by its own intelligence. It enters a dormant stage, sometimes forever, sometimes re-emerging in a midlife crisis, in the experience of having a child, in facing death or one of its symbolic equivalents.

We psychotherapists live with patterns of passive acceptance of patient and community demands, which if not countered, lead to self-destruction or paralysis. Psychotherapy patterns turn into "schools" which escape passivity by turning to models with prescribed behavioral sequences, or by seeking validation in science with a data-base from which inevitable conclusions may be derived (Keith & Whitaker, 1978).

All of these models (model = myth without divine characters) inhibit

David V. Keith, M.D., is in practice with the Family Therapy Institute, Inc., 790 So. Cleveland Avenue, St. Paul, MN 55116. He is Adjunct Associate Professor, Department of Family Social Science, University of Minnesota, Minneapolis.

spontaneous behavior by therapists with the implied threat of damage to patients. The structure which develops as a protective cage for the Self of the therapist comes to dominate and frustrate the therapist. While the patients of the imprisoned therapist remain undamaged, many continue to have a problem. They can make social changes, but do not gain personal spontaneity.

If the therapist cannot be a self, neither can the patient. It is my recurring belief that if the therapist remains in a professional role, the patient is unable to leave the complementary role. The model for the role-dominated patient is the good child, socially adapted, but without imagination.

If the therapist cannot be a self, neither the can client [handwritten margin note]

There is a well-worn, but illustrative, joke about an old psychiatrist and a young psychiatrist getting on the elevator at the end of a day's work. The old psychiatrist is fresh-looking, immaculately groomed with a carnation in his lapel. The young psychiatrist is disheveled and tired-looking. He says to his older colleague, "How do you listen to this stuff all day, and come out looking so fresh?" Says the old psychiatrist, "Who listens?" The old psychiatrist is all professional role and each day is a carbon copy of the one preceding.

The problem for the therapist is how to make a Houdini-like escape from the chains of professional image and survive. That is where the person of the therapist comes in. Because, for better or for worse, the dynamics of therapy are in the person of the therapist (Whitaker & Malone, 1953). And while the Self cannot be "known" in an assured, left-brained, take-a-final-examination-way, it needs to be familiar so that the mature professional therapist can guide it.

It is important to note that the author works as a family therapist. Therefore, the focus is on the *interpersonal* components of health and pathology. Likewise, implicit in the paper is that this personal self is best known in relation to other selves, for our purposes here, cotherapists and patients. These ideas do not translate automatically into individual therapy patterns. The personal self is much more suspect in working with individuals. The presence of the family and the cotherapist allows more freedom and security for patients and therapists. An exception would be when a cotherapy team works with an individual.

In the midst of writing, my wife, Noel, and I visited an art museum. We were standing back admiring one of Jackson Pollock's giant paintings. "See if you can find any form in that canvas," says Noel. I could not. "Now, fix on a dot, and see if you can hold it." I could not. The dynamic, fluid quality of Pollock's work did not offer any specific form nor would it allow the eye to rest. It demanded movement. Noel said, "That's the way your paper comes across. It is interesting, but it is sometimes difficult to . . . . . " That story is a guide to your involvement with this paper. The suggestion that my thinking was patternless and confused was a little hurtful, but I enjoyed the comparison to Jackson Pollock.

This personal Self of the therapist is, in fact, a community of selves. The mayor of this community is the professional self. It has a professional degree, does diagnostic interviews, maintains technical proficiency, reads professional journals, and takes few chances. The subject of this paper is a more obscure self, the personal Self; the one that would rather be on the floor building a Lego spaceship with the four-year-old, than writing this paper.

This personal Self with its capital "S" is something we experience obliquely, understand with our peripheral vision and see through a glass but darkly. It sneaks up on us. It is unintentional. It did not decide to become a Self. It did not decide to be conceived. It began with an orgastic communion of selves, and is best known by its appearance in interpersonal experience. It also appears in dream experience, unexpectedly and often inscrutably.

This elusive Self with its capital "S" is something I have forever wanted to know. But "know" is the wrong word. In my 5th decade "familiar" rings more true. I am familiar with my Self to the point of being both pleased and pained with its familiar unpredictability. In dreams it appears as a giant in a miniature world, as a lover, as a woman, and as a bare-fisted warrior. Sometimes the Self is helpless and fleeing, sometimes it is confused and often partially dressed. Oddly, its occasional appearances in therapy metaphorically mirror the dream appearances.

This Self is crazy and creative. Often, it is too playful for its own good. And it strains to speak or to appear with eccentric overtones. Its intuitive accuracy sometimes surprises. This self has no firm image. It is that furtive schizophrenic, both chronic and acute, fragmented and out of focus. It forgets to return certain phone calls, and negatively hallucinates most administrative responsibilities. It has a certain Christ-like quality, hungry to change the world, too often thinking of death as just another dream possibility from which it will awaken. In its hunger for love and other variations of human contact, it is impetuous and frequently shows poor judgement. Its simultaneous arrogance and humility leads to silence. Flickers of rage appear at the edges. Haunted by dependency, it looks furtively backward at the ghost of failure.

But this Self is not just a Me. It is an amalgam of endless fragments from those deeply loved. I am most apt to find It in relation to someone else. I often wonder, am I really a me or just a complicated sum of my relationships? "Did I just say that, or was it one of those fragments speaking out of turn?"

During a difficult period in a struggle I was having with a family, the father remarked, speaking of psychotherapy, "I can never understand how they get intelligent people to do this kind of work." There are times when I feel the same way. But, what he could not see, and what I often forget, is the seductive quality that therapy with families has. Nor could he see how often I am able to leave my therapist's chair and become a patient with the deep pleasure of contacting another Self in those indescribable moments of bilateral therapeutic experience.

SOME FEATURES OF THE PERSONAL SELF

This is a preliminary exploration on a series of notes kept over the past 8 years; a view of the Self from a therapist's sketchbook, if you will. For all I know there may be no such thing. The Self which may be spoken of, is not the true Self. It may be only like the unicorn, a mythical beast. Or like the Adult, it may exist only as a theoretical construct. What is crucial is its availability in relation to the Other.

The Self appears by surprise. When it appears, the professional self decides whether to recognize It. Although there are those moments when It either bursts or sneaks, in circumventing protocol. It is there during an awkward moment in therapy; one that we wished had not happened. But then a therapeutic shift is noticed at the next interview. Sometimes in the evening, at home, my family hears me groan or sees me shake my head. It usually means that I am having a flashback to a family therapy session and something I said or failed to say. It probably also means that the Self found its way into the session. Those flashbacks happen rarely, if at all, in relation to sessions with individuals.

For better or for worse, this Self is:

— Against the culture. It is the part of us which is not socially-adapted.
— Creative or crazy or spontaneous and unpredictable.
— Often ridiculous or silly.
— Largely unconscious.
-- Potentially dangerous to me as well as to the other. It is not convinced that death really means anything.
— Often ridiculous.
— Inconsistent.
— Not anesthetized by "born-again" enthusiasm, but struggles with the pain of growing until death comes.

THE SELF AS IT APPEARS IN THERAPY

The following are some manifestations of the Self as it appears in therapy. What is coming into focus is that the therapist's personal Self appears only in relation to the patient's personal Self.

— Power.
— Integrity.
— Sense of my absurdity and the use of humor.

— Freedom for anger and creative hatred.
— Metaphorical reality.
— Residue of outside experiences.
— Freedom to advance or retreat from any position (Whitaker, 1976).
— Development of peer relationships (Cotherapy).
— Ability to be freely loving.

Power

Bateson has protested the use of physics concepts, like power, for de-scribing human relationships (Keeney, 1983, p. 125). I am always uneasy in disagreeing with Bateson, but the etymology of power has to do with human behavior, which is inescapably cybernetic, meaning "to be able" (Partridge, 1958). In therapy, I link power with the freedom to use my professional image or to be myself, at my initiative. I consider it a limited freedom.

In the beginning of therapy, power has to do with the freedom to set the structure for the therapy. Who will be there, when and where will we meet? In the first interview, power has to do with how the information will be presented. This component is managed by the professional self.

At the second interview the professional self continues to dominate. Power is used to stay out. "What do you want from me? Are you certain you want to be here? Maybe we should quit now." There is a serious question about who shall provide motivation for family change, the thera-pist or the family's desperation. Palazzoli (1985) asks, "Why do patients make it so hard for us to help them?" Too often the professional assumes that because they made an appointment, they want to be in therapy. Often, they come in only to see what is needed. Before the next step is taken, they need to sign the operative permit. The professional often urges that therapy continue. They make it hard for us to help them be-cause we take away the family's responsibility for itself. The Self of the patient with its intuition warns of hidden danger.

There is a good example of this problem in the way that child psychia-try is sometimes practiced. Too often, child psychiatrists believe that they can parent better than the real parents. The child psychiatry version of family therapy has the quality of child psychiatry training for the parents. Parents learn to be professional. As I think of family therapy it offers an opportunity for the family to have the therapeutically valuable, regressive experience of patienthood.

As caring increases, power diminishes or equalizes in the relationship context (Keith, 1981). At this point it is not possible to push families around. The fluctuating dance of therapy begins as the therapist moves in and out, close in with caring and attention, then distant and indifferent. Now the power of the therapist resides in the capacity to change himself, the power to join and the power to separate. The mode is similar to parenting, where the mother has the freedom to shift generational level as needed. She may sometimes be parental. "Before you go ride your bike you are going to clean your room." At other times she is a peer. "Let's make rhubarb pie and surprise Dad." Or she may be a generation down. "Do you think I'm being unfair?" Power is manifested in the capacity to move between generations rather than moving in response to the other's demand.

Integrity

Technical proficiency is the professional precursor of integrity. Integrity colors decision-making, and can bring us into conflict with the community. As experience accumulates, the demands on the professional self may be in conflict with the demands of the personal self. An example would be a psychiatrist who grows uncomfortable with the use of psychotropic medication and the community expectations for a psychiatrist.

Integrity of the Self refuses to become any image that is offered. The doctor part of me is a role function. I am not a physician, I work as a physician.

Integrity does not permit the Self to presume to know what the Other thinks. Likewise, it does not permit Other to think they know what Self thinks.

Integrity refuses to be all knowing and is comfortable with the knowledge that all human problems do not have answers.

Sense of My Absurdity and the Use of Humor

I like humor and find it useful in working with families. It is always spontaneous, and with adults the most available form of play therapy. Psychotherapy takes place in the overlap of two areas of playing, that of the therapist and that of the patient (Winnicott, 1971).

Humor can have a sadistic and distancing quality, but what is hidden is the way it introduces sudden moments of intimacy and peer relationship. Humor by itself is not sadistic, it is the *person* who is sadistic. Humor by itself is not distancing, it is the person that is distancing. There are times after an interview which has had a feeling of fun and intimacy, when I will feel vaguely depressed. It must be because of the loneliness that follows closeness. So in that sense, humor makes us aware of the distance in our relationships or of the sadistic components that lie beneath that thin veneer of social protocol.

Humor distorts reality and allows us to see another way, exploding the bonds of logic or social propriety. For example, when the 13-year-old son was rude to the 45-year-old therapist, the father scolded him, saying that he "should show more respect to Dr. . . . " He could not remember the doctor's name. "Just call me 'Butch,'" said the therapist.

Humor acts as a wonderful enzyme for making the symptom interpersonal. Telling a joke, using double entendre or a gentle tease is an ambiguous invitation to be personal. Shared humor is a self-to-self experience.

Humor is a way to be insulting without being annihilating. The therapeutic relationship may induce an anesthetized infantalism in the patient if the therapist is too supportive. Gentle insults induce individuation with concommitant self-responsibility.

The following case sample illustrates. The Fakes were referred by the pediatrician because their previously angelic daughter, age 14, had evidenced mild disobedience. The father was passive and lethargic. The mother was neurotic and hyperactive. She mentioned being on a medication which she referred to as her "sleeping dope." The cotherapists took it to be a reference to her husband.

By the way, How many family therapists does it take to change a light bulb? Forget the light bulb, let's rewire the house.

Did you hear about the Norwegian who loved his wife so much he almost told her?

Humor is like any spice. It must be infused in right proportion so as to improve the taste. Beware using humor to depersonalize therapeutic experience. A symptom may be the therapist's anxiety mounting before adding the humor. In fact, anxiety in the therapist may be a specific contradiction to using humor. Finally, humor can turn into an empty runaway, nonsense with no affective implications.

Freedom for Anger and Creative Hatred

If you have not been hated by your therapist, you have been cheated (Winnicott, 1949). Anger and hatred are ways to be more deeply interpersonal. To extrapolate from Winnicott, if there is no hatred there is no marriage. And are our children cheated when we fail to hate them?

In this era of self-understanding and conscious efforts at parenting, we learn we should not come down to our children's level. That is, we should not be as hateful toward them as they are to us. Yet, if we seal ourselves off they are cheated and burdened by the illusion that anger and hatred are personally inappropriate. Therapists are like parents. When the therapist comes down to their level, both grow from it when the generation gap is reestablished.

Case Example

Working with Mrs. L, a chronic mental patient, and her grown daughter over a period of a year was both frustrating and satisfying. As she left the life of chronic mental patient and became more self-owning she began a pattern of admiring her therapist in a way which he found increasingly aggravating. His frustration mounted one day as she went on and on about him, until he exploded, "Will you shut up! Just shut up!" She was insulted and left saying she would not return. After she left, the therapist was remorseful, but felt it best that the situation be allowed to take its own course. Mrs. T returned three weeks later. In effect she had ended therapy and now restarted. She said that while she had been initially insulted it occurred to her that her esteemed doctor may be having a nervous breakdown. If he, an esteemed doctor was having a nervous breakdown, it somehow made her history more human.

Metaphorical Reality

This is the most creative component of any therapy, it is that jointly unconscious poetry, that moves in and out of awareness. It is found in our verbal slips, in the adjective which we hear ourselves using with this particular family, or in visual images stimulated by their presence.

Children live constantly in this reality. I am suspicious of families and therapists who think they do more "work" by leaving the children home. The children's presence enriches the metaphorical atmosphere of therapy, which increases the likelihood of the whole person being affected by the experience.

John Sonne's (1973) concept of the Metaphorolytic family has been useful to me. This is a family which allows experience to have only one level of meaning. This is the kind of family that does not know how to play, the kind of family that is cornered by its own normality.

Case Sample

The Drs. H., a psychologist and an economist, struggled in their marriage. Both were paralyzed by their professional images. She became extensively self-mutilating and he increasingly distant and work preoccupied. Their 4-year-old daughter was present in the interviews which the therapists video-taped. The H's asked to see a videotaped interview, but watched only a short segment, complaining that the noise their daughter created as she played made it impossible to hear the adult conversation. When the therapist looked at the tape, the daughter was playing a game with dolls. Her "noise" was the doll crying, "Help, mama. Mama help. Somebody help her." The recording of her play was the most crucial subtext of the interview, giving voice to her mother's anguish. But the parents in their effort to be more realistic (metaphorolytic) about the problem heard only non-metaphorical noise.

Residue of Outside Experience

The psychotherapy koan, the dynamics of therapy are in the person of the therapist (Whitaker & Malone, 1953) suggest that the therapist's outside living dynamics feed the therapy situation. If outside living is dead, is the therapist's effectiveness diminished? There are those times when the therapist is disrupted by events in personal life; a child is ill, the therapists marriage is disrupted. These real-life troubles may alter functioning, but not necessarily in a detrimental way. Often while technical proficiency diminishes, the Person is more present.

At a time when we were preparing to move to another city, I began to think of moving as a symbolic death. It was impressive how often death became an issue in the families I was working with.

In reviewing my psychotherapeutic work with schizophrenics I developed a list of schizophrenic patients with whom I had had profound experiences. I was impressed to discover that each one corresponded with periods of personal emotional arousal. Four were time-related to the birth of our children and another to a time when I was a psychotherapy patient.

The Freedom to Advance or Retreat from Any Position

The Self is not paralyzed by reason or consistency. It changes hypotheses so that any problem can be seen from a different perspective. It is available to see unexpected change in a family. The freedom to be inconsistent is another doorway to creativity for the family. At one point in the interview the Self may empathically support the scapegoat's effort to change the family, then later tease him for being a boor. No family becomes a fixed theoretical construct.

The Development of Peer Relationships

The split image (therapist/person) is most available in an experienced cotherapy connection that permits creative craziness in the therapy interview without meta-processing.

Likewise, the self of the patients is more present when their family is present.

The Capacity to be Freely Loving

Developing the capacity to be freely loving is a primary goal of psychotherapy. It emerges with experience, lies out beyond the realm of technique, and requires the balanced functioning of the professional and the personal selves.

Of interest to me as I work on the concept of the Self in the therapist is how often my experience as a patient returns, I recall hearing our therapist say that he loved me, but I did not believe it for a long time. When I did I ended being a patient. Our patients need to know that we love them. In that way they can begin to give up being patients.

SUMMARY

This personal Self speaks in half truths and innuendo. Thus most of what is included here is only partially true and should not be translated directly into the reader's experience.

The professional self, a social role, provides the structure for the personal Self to make appearances in family therapy. This Self does not show up as a free standing entity, but rather as part of a joint experience with the Self that lies behind the patient self, another social role. The therapist's Self appears as an invitation to the patient's Self to appear. An important result of the communion of selves is in the joy of acknowledging another Self, but satisfied with the fact that they are separate. In successful therapy they end as peers.

And the Self lived everafter, however, not always happily.

BIBLIOGRAPHY

Keeney, B.P. (1983). *Aesthetics of change*. New York: The Guilford Press.
Keith, D.V. (1981). Power: Physical or mental? A response. *Pilgrimage*, 9, 32-33.
Keith, D.V. & Whitaker, C.A. (1978, January). Struggling with the impotence impasse: Absurdity and acting in. *Journal of marital and family counseling*, 69-77.
Palazzoli-Selvini, M. (1985, October). Towards a general model of psychotic family games. Address presented at the 43rd Annual Conference, American Association of Marital and Family Therapists, New York.
Partridge, E. (1958). *Origins, a short etymological dictionary of modern english*. New York: Macmillan Publishing Company, Inc.
Sonne, J. (1973). *A primer for family therapists*. Moorestown, NJ: The Thursday Press.
Whitaker, C.A. (1976). The hindrance of theory in clinical work. In P. Guerin (Ed.) *Family therapy: Theory and practice*. New York: Gardner Press.
Whitaker, C.A. & Malone, T.P. (1953). *The roots of psychotherapy*. New York: Blakiston Press.
Winnicot, D.W. (1949). Hate in the countertransference. International journal of psychoanalysis, 30, 69-74.
Winnicott, D.W. (1971). *Playing and Reality*. New York: Basic Books.

Uses of the Self
in Integrated Contextual
Systems Therapy

Bunny S. Duhl

ABSTRACT. In this article, the author discusses some of the generic ways in which she regards use of the self important, implying that certain processes in training can attend to this development in trainees. Drawing upon anecdotes from her personal life, she then demonstrates how she uses her learnings to intervene in therapy situations. The author also describes how through using herself spatially and physically, both therapist and clients can obtain systemic views of relationships and create new ways of thinking and acting.

How do I use myself in therapy?* To paraphase Elizabeth Barrett Browning, "Let me count the ways." As a family systems therapist, I draw on everything I have ever experienced, learned or done in this life which connects me to myself and other human beings. I use my awareness and my learnings about how we think, image, feel, experience, act, understand, grow and change. In addition to more "formal education," I draw analogs from my experience as a musician, a flutist, in my awareness of how different "instruments" can be in rhythm, harmonize, or be discordant. As a potter and sculptor for some 20 years, I draw upon a wealth of processes and images, and the knowledge that the same "material" can take many different forms, and that something that never existed before can evolve and take shape, when handled "correctly." A delightful series of experiences in theatre from an early age through college summer stock definitely provided a way later of seeing family systems and supported the idea that one could play many roles as both

Bunny S. Duhl, Ed.D., is Co-Director of the Boston Family Institute. She may be reached at 55 Williston Road, Brookline, MA 02146.

*For ease, novelty, and in this case, personal preference, I have chosen to use the pronoun "her" and "herself" for therapist rather than the usual him/herself awkward phrase. No gender prejudice is meant.

71

family member as well as therapist. I constantly draw on that sense of family as theatre (Duhl, 1983). In my experience as a writer, I draw upon the challenge, as now, to zero in on that which is holographic and translate it into linear language in ways that hopefully communicate to others. I most certainly draw upon my experience as woman, wife, mother of three children, daughter, sister and orphan. Especially, I draw upon my awareness of being a woman at this particular time in history with my own experiences of changing roles, values, expectations, opportunities and lifestyles.

So how do I use myself in therapy? In as many ways as I possibly can which allow me to tune into that which matters to each person, and that which will help support the transformation of pain into option, problem into creative solution, and "stuckness" into movement, with the tools for further understanding and movement in the hands of each client.

AN INTEGRATED CONTEXTUAL SYSTEMS MODEL

The model of working with people to which I subscribe is an integrated contextual systems model, with a base in family therapy (Duhl & Duhl, 1981). This family therapy systems model essentially derives from general systems (von Bertalanffy, 1968) and learning theory (Piaget, 1952; in Gruber & Voneche, 1977). The constructs and concepts of social and family systems interactions are cross cut with individual and family developmental models, with great emphasis on how our minds work at each age and stage, and on how learning-to-learn takes place in varying contexts (Duhl & Duhl, 1981). Developed at the Boston Family Institute since 1969 (Duhl & Duhl, 1974, 1979; Duhl, 1983, 1986), this particular model focusses on the human capacity for meaning making and the search for coherence. Each of us as human beings makes sense of the world as best we can, given the developmental cognitive stages through which we wend our way and the totality of the contexts in which we are embedded. This model is also cognizant of the miraculous human capacity to believe those products of our own minds—the meanings we ourselves have made—AS IF they constitute the ultimate and only truth about each situation we have encountered and pondered.

Change in this integrated contextual systems model is seen as deriving from internal and external reconfigurations. Internally, helping people *to update the way in which they hold beliefs, meanings and information*, through some form of reframing, allows them to experience themselves in a new relationship to that information. Externally, helping people *to experience and enact alternative ways of behaving and relating* allows them to experience a different relationship to others. Both aspects are necessary for lasting change (Bateson, 1979). Transforming beliefs and behaviors requires offering optional images and metaphors for those which seem to bind people in fear of the unknown—whether that unknown be the next stage in their lives (Andolfi et al., 1983) or a way of living without fear. Perhaps the most important task in the change process a therapist encounters is tuning people into their own rich resources which have not yet been tapped and offering them tools with which to use these resources in daily life and problem solving.

The Roles of the Therapist

While in such a model, the "client" may be a couple, a family, the total important network, or even one person, the role of the therapist in her use of self in totality, is *to safeguard and promote the autonomy of each person's fluid interconnection with others.* The therapist knows that each person influences and is influenced by each other person in the system (von Bertalanffy, 1968), and that each has a personal and idiosyncratic view of issues and events. Each person's view adds a dynamic to the whole. Each is correct, none is complete. The therapist herself has another view, that of how all members interact in her presence, which allows for a view of how the total family system functions in patterned ways (Duhl, 1983). Since no one view is complete, the contextual systems therapist must not be bound and bonded to any one individual in a family or extended personal group, but must use herself in a mobile way so as to be able to "stand behind" each person in the room while seeing the patterns, both flexible and blocked, that interactions among individuals create.

When a therapist is with a family, she uses herself in multiple roles (Satir, 1972a). As an empathic listener, she validates each person's view of events. As an artful "dodge'em car" operator, she carefully maneuvers between "obstacles," notably the persons in the family who insist their view is the only correct one. In reflecting to the family the patterns that are repetitive, she acts as a mirror highlighting that which they cannot see themselves. She is an improvisational theatre director as she asks family members to enact new ways of relating to each other, or places them in motion in a sculptural spatial metaphor of change (Duhl, Kantor & Duhl, 1973; Duhl, 1983). Much of the time she is a weaver, linking images, behaviors, thoughts, and experiences with context, and connecting all in a textured tapestry of life.

In the instance where the client is one individual with a contextual systems therapist, the therapist particularly uses herself as historian, anthropologist, and dramatist. In these roles, the therapist is seeking and gathering information concerning contexts and other people with whom the client is and has been connected. She needs to generate the "map" of the total system and its interactional nature for both herself, and for the client. When she has that "map," she is able to promote those optional behaviors, thoughts, feelings, beliefs that fit the situation and the particular individuals involved, so that new possibilities can take form.

Within a contextual systems model, input from so-called outsiders such as relatives, agencies, teachers, is not only accepted but desired. Through multiple inputs, the therapist can understand not only the interactional shaping impacts each person has on each other, but can understand the way in which each person "holds" others in his mind—in his emotions and symbolic meanings. Thus the contextual systems therapist knows that to help create fluidity where there were blockages within an individual as well as between people, to understand the way in which symptoms play a part in the play of life, she as therapist must also be a detective and playwright. Listening and imaging with dramatic flair, the therapist then is involved in mentally fleshing out the cast of characters with each in his specific roles, replete with lines and actions as well as each one's idiosyncratic way of being in and perceiving the world. Grasping how others construct and hold their realities offers the therapist the routes of access for introducing alternative and equally viable constructions (Minuchin, 1974; Watzlawick et al., 1974).

Using oneself as therapist then with this model means first to know oneself well, to know the meanings one harbours, and where and when they come from. It also means to be a cartographer and biographer of each person in the room—to know each person, understanding how each has made his meanings of interactive process, given the influences of family beliefs, ethnic and contextual background, and developmental time. It means to care about the people one sees, yet not to get caught in that caring.

IMPLICATIONS FOR THE TRAINEE AND TRAINING

How one arrives at being able to do these types of mental schematics is a matter of the type of education—drawing forth, in which each trainee learning to become a therapist immerses herself. Within such a training model as the one developed at the Boston Family Institute, it is necessary for the future therapist to become aware of the systems within the self as well as between persons. In that process, it is equally necessary that she be free (as were the pioneers in the field) to use all of her own life experiences to draw upon. This means in training, heightening the awareness of one's way of thinking and believing at each stage of life in order to rekindle that which has been dormant. Appreciating the idiosyncratic styles we each have of processing information, and their fit with how we expected ourselves to learn, and our feelings about ourselves, becomes as important as how different learning styles and stages fit together in one family (Duhl & Duhl, 1975; Duhl, 1983, 1986).

To be cognizant of a wide frame within which to work with families means to explore the myths, rules and binds that hold families together, one's own as well as others, to examine the stories and core images one has of one's family and other strangers, to explore and play with the myriad ways family members interact while handling their vulnerabilities and defenses (Duhl, 1976). When we each as trainee investigate the ways in which we hook others into our schemes and get hooked into theirs, we have some sense of approximation of what might also be going on for clients. Approximation is the closest we will ever get to knowing how another experiences the world. The more we each know about ourselves and the others with whom we learn, the more we can know and move with that which is generic in all persons. To be free to use oneself means to recognize many ways that loving, playing, fighting, deciding, mourning, can happen and to know that each person in life is busy trying to maintain his sense of self esteem (Satir, 1964, 1972b) while going towards imaged goals in a world each never made.

Using oneself fully means to know patterns of clear and muddy communication in one's own systems as well as those one works with and within (Satir, 1964; Watzlawick et al., 1967). Considering the boundaries in one's family, and all the ways those boundaries manifested themselves, takes trainees into looking at family rules, roles, routines and replications (Duhl & Duhl, 1979). Use of self requires oneself as trainee and as therapist to continually update one's life, while examining oneself as an actor in the systems one is in (Anonymous, 1972).

Using oneself well then means to be involved in an ongoing research project: to be curious about one's own reactions and intentions in varying contexts, and to locate the source of reactivity in one's learned-to-learn patterns. These patterns, developed in earlier contexts, give clues to the current context as well as the context of clients. Such a model implies the continual development of one's capacity to respond creatively in life situations as well as in therapy, to be in touch with one's existential core in relation to one's life in context at each period of time. It means to play with options for oneself, with a wide range of stances and roles from which to choose. Then one has many creative ways to invent metaphor, humor, and ways of making the familiar strange and the strange familiar (Gordon & Poze, 1973). Most of all, over time, it means to trust oneself—to be able to reach inside and know how to tune into the inner core of oneself en route to other persons, and to know that to be human is to unfold and conserve in varying degrees at different times.

Many ways of specifically describing oneself as therapist are possible.

I will focus here on interventions drawn from life experience, and inventions in clinical practice, hopefully stimulating readers to consider what each brings to her practice drawn from life or spontaneously created. After all, one person's invention becomes another's "technique."

PROBLEM-SOLVING ANECDOTES: INTERVENTIONS FROM MY LIFE

One's own style as person obviously is the core of one's style as therapist. I seem to be one of those people who is both experimental and introspective in life, particularly about actions taken with others. I have often experimented with, "what if I did this?" and "what if I tried that?" and to record in my mind the results of new experimental behaviors. I did that in my work with clay, and with my interactions with people. In addition, long before I was a family therapist, when in a pickle, and some unplanned and spontaneous action or response on my part also seemed to "work" to untangle an interactive knot, I later would think about the sequences and underlying constructs of such action, and figure out why such actions made a difference in the system. Naturally, this style of being enters into my world as a contextual systems therapist. Thus, over my lifetime, I have built up a large personal repertoire of problem-solving responses to which I continually add, which are often useful in my integrated contextual systems approach to client's situations.

The Clean-Up Fight

There are certain generic issues in families, which also have concomitant generic behavioral patterns around them. When families are into a repetitive fighting style involving parents and young teenagers particularly, around cleaning up rooms or doing household tasks, I often use this first anecdote.

When our son was about 12, I had been after him for several days to clean up his gear in the playroom-TV room. Each time I asked him, or told him to do it, he said he would get around to it, and of course, didn't. We were into a repetitive cycle that went nowhere, each time doing "more of the same" (Watzlawick et al., 1974).

On the fourth or fifth day, when I'd "had it" with his lack of action, I entered the room when he was in it and no longer asked, but commanded him to clean it up. He, equally strident in voice tone, said he would get to it. I raised my voice. He raised his. I raised mine. Again, he raised his. And than I caught something and went up the scale in tone. He went up higher—and this continued until we both were squeaking at each other and burst out laughing. The room was cleaned up within a half hour. We had each vented our annoyance, mine at his not listening, and he at being told what to do. In addition, we had interrupted the repetitive cycle in which we were both involved in a way that allowed for a win-win result.

Uses of This Story

I use this story in several ways: the first use is empathic—as a way of helping a family to feel more at ease and safe to take risks, by using myself as an example of system member who was in an ordinary family bind, and who got out of it. I emphasize the spontaneity of my noticing something and making a conscious decision to act differently—that is, to "play" in the middle of a fight, by going up a tone of the scale. I also emphasize my son 's willingness to "play," indicating that often the other party in a stuck cycle is also looking for a new way out. One must be open to switching gears, particularly when one is annoyed, to turn blame into a win-win face-saving situation.

A second way in which I use this anecdote is as the model for my intervention. I suggest that for a week, family members are to have this kind of angry exchange whenever they fight, with each one yelling his point of view and then literally escalating the tone till squeaking is reached. Such a prescription enacted puts people in a different relationship to their anger, their fights, and each other. It takes them out of the justified, self righteous ego position with which we are all familiar, and frees them to be more flexible and forgiving of self and others. In interrupting the automatic style of fighting, participants become actively conscious of their own repetitive patterns and the novelty of new ones.

A third usage is as an example of doing something different with a repeated fight—with the suggestion that they are to find something else different and humorous to do with their "automatic pilot" fights, which will allow for a win-win situation. Their own creativity is sparked, tapping unused resources (Minuchin, 1974). By changing their actions, family members often become clearer concerning what else the fight has stood for.

A fourth way in which I use this is to empower children to be able to be angry, to vent anger, without it being seen as disrespectful and forbidden. Suggesting such a structure for fighting creates an arena for both parent and child to play their roles fully AND to arrive at a different balance in their relationship both to self and with each other.

Ritual Roles with Children

Again, in the service of letting clients know that their "stuck places" are places all of us as parents have been in, I will share an anecdote of major importance to me in my life which has become a reusable generic systemic intervention for me with myself as well as with clients.

About 6 years ago, when our youngest daughter was about 15, I found myself in a peculiar place with her, where we would get into some kind of repeated tangle as I listened to her tales of woe, of "what went wrong in school today." I would try to help her sort what was going on. Each time I would start out open, feel sympathetic, listen, offer a comment, only to find her objecting and defensive, with whatever I said. I then would get more entangled, enquiring WHY she was defensive. She became even more so, and I felt annoyed and frustrated. Of course I tried to get HER to change! and be "reasonable," which went nowhere. We were into a repetitive loop that I began to dread. And then one day, I realized that I was bored with myself, with my own "tape recordings," and I made one rule of thumb for myself: *that whatever I said or did in relation to her around these repetitive situations, it would be something I had never said or done before!* Now there was an interesting challenge! *I would switch my focus to my part* of this continuing loop.

The very next day after school she came to talk to me with her latest "sad" story. I quickly remembered my promise to myself and braced for the unexpected. I did not know what I would come up with. After her opening comment, I looked at her, smiled and said, "Gee your eyes are pretty today." She looked startled and went on talking. I then said, "Your hair looks nice too. Did you do something different with it?" At this point she started to complain, almost whining, "Mommmm, you're not listening!" At which point, because I almost started to giggle, I looked out the window and commented on the two squirrels who were chasing each other. She got annoyed. And I kept up my end of the non-hooked dialogue. I was irrelevant, irreverent, silly, absurd. I can't even remember after those first few interchanges what I said. All I know is that I kept myself from saying anything I'd ever said before. She slammed out of the room and I smiled, licked my thumb and gave myself a "medal" on my chest with it. I felt excited. I hadn't gotten into any "tape recorded" dialogue.

The second day a similar event took place and this time when she went out of the room she not only slammed the door with an "I don't know what's the matter with you!", but she swore at me as well—enough to trigger me to start out of my chair, angry. Half way up I caught myself and realized *this was only the next level of hooking me into her issues* and into tangling with her in the old angry way. And so I sat down again, smiled and once more felt triumphant and excited.

The third time she came to talk to me about her daily miseries and I said I particularly liked what she was wearing, she stopped to look and to comment nicely that she liked it too. And as she again went into her story and I said something absurd, she laughed and countered with something tentatively funny. And I knew we were off the dime and into a new dialogue as she began to lighten up, and talk about her day in a different way.

Our dialogues have been different ever since, for it takes at least two to make a repetitive interactional pattern. The success of this "intervention" on my own pattern at that time is strong reinforcement whenever I find myself in such "loops" with anyone. I use it to get unhooked again.

The Elements for "Success"

As I thought about this long and hard afterwards, I realized that there were several elements in what I had done that ensured success, which I had not thought about when I decided to "do something different":

The main element relates to the fact that when one person changes their side of a known script or pattern and holds to that change, the other person MUST change too in order to maintain any kind of connection (Bowen, 1978; Watzlawick et al., 1974).

In terms of the success of the type of change of dialogue on my part, the opening comments I made to her were positive and about her person. My focus was on HER and I was paying attention to HER, *not* what she was saying. The comments were made with genuine appreciation for I had chosen things about her I liked each time. It seemed to work as a confusionary set of statements for she had a hard time getting annoyed with my positive attributions about her person.

A third element relates to my voice tone which stayed light and interested in whatever I was talking about, which of course, was everything BUT her "problem." This too was confusionary. The paraverbal message conveyed interest. The content message conveyed disinterest in the problem (Watzlawick et al., 1967). She could not react in her ordinary way to this new noncongruent communication, and therefore had to switch the total communication pattern in a type of second order change (Watzlawick et al., 1974).

The fourth element here, one of functional autonomy, was in my personal agenda not to be bored with myself and therefore not to get hooked, which took primacy over everything else. The sense of delight in my own agenda allowed me to be absurd, and stay free. It certainly beat feeling frustrated!

Yet another element was not to buy into the next level of hooking—that of her swearing. I stayed constant in my irrelevance to her behavior. That in itself meant that her conversation with me would have to change, if indeed she were to continue to want to talk to me anymore. It was a risk I was willing to take, based on the amount and type of connection we already had.

Lastly, I had already learned that one needs an "N" of at least 3 experiences with anything new in one's life in order to begin to have a sense of pattern and of change (Duhl, 1983). The first time around is experience itself. One has never been there before and you can't know ahead of time what exactly will happen or what it will feel like. The second time around with any type of experience allows for comparison. This situation is like that one, or is not like that one. The third time around one has the opportunity for observing a pattern—that events will fall into one or another category or become yet a third category, in which case one can begin to look for the pattern of categories from the third experience on. And so with this situation, I knew we would need AT LEAST 3 go-arounds to begin to get a flavor of what would happen to change our previous ritual hooking pattern.

Uses of This Anecdote

This particular story I tell to families and to individuals—to parents without their children present, and sometimes to children without their parents present if they are old enough to comprehend and carry out such behavior. I tell it to wives without husbands present and husbands seen without wives, and to adult children trying to deal with their siblings, friends, and parents. In short, I will use it in multiple situations where *being hooked* is the issue. I call being hooked "the Velcro effect." There is "negative Velcro" and "positive Velcro." "Negative Velcro" is any repeated pattern where participants end up feeling defeated, incompetent, with concomitant low self esteem. "Positive Velcro" loops are mutually enhancing growth allowing patterns.

With clients I zero in on and reframe the real issue as one of boredom—being bored with oneself. I suggest that one might as well have a good time and some adventure, since the ongoing repeated dialogue doesn't seem to be much fun. I stress the agenda of the personal triumph of novelty and that it is to be a secret. I suggest focussing positively first on the person of the other, and that after that, anything is fair game as long as the tone is light, cheerful, as if one were with a wonderful companion on an outing. The imagery I try to evoke is filled with pleasure. I prepare people for the flak of change as I tell them the more flak there is, the more you know you are being successful (Bowen, 1978). I warn them that the "opponent" will probably try to escalate the game with the next level of hooking, like my daughter's swearing, and that they must be on guard not to fall into the trap.

A Clinical Example

Recently, I was seeing a mother and her 28-year-old daughter who were caught in their version of "negative Velcro" loops, each complaining about the other and each wanting something of the other pertinent to much earlier developmental stages for each of them. The daughter had been working sporadically as a waitress for almost a year, though formerly capable of managerial positions, and wanted mother to "give" to her. Mother wanted the daughter to continue to seek and heed her advice and standards. Each was afraid of the next stage in their lives. They were now living separately. I saw the mother alone one time, told her this anecdote and focussed on her boredom and frustration. She agreed. She was to adopt this method with her daughter. When I next saw them, the mother sat smiling as her daughter complained that she "wasn't the old mother that she used to be," and that she "wanted her old mother back." Mother remained unhooked. Shortly after that, the daughter reported that she had begun looking for a new job, more equivalent to her skills, which she subsequently found. While this was not the sole intervention in my work with this dyad, it was the first major dislocator of the negative Velcro loop.

In so many interpersonal situations, DOING SOMETHING DIFFERENT with *oneself* is the key to changing self AND context, yet it often feels like heavy duty bad medicine. I personally prefer humor as a vehicle of change, for it feels like an adding on rather than a giving up of behavior, and indeed it is. However, the more one adds on, the less room and time there is for "old" behavior, and the more fun one is having in the process (Duhl & Duhl, 1981).

ONE-PERSON SCULPTURE FLESHED OUT

In another way of using myself, this time, physically, I often do a family sculpture with one person (Duhl, 1983) when other family members are not in the area. The first time I did this years ago, the 33-year-old Southern woman I started seeing reported that she had always been depressed. I wanted to get a picture of the interactional context in which she had grown up.

I had my client enact each family member first, while I momentarily stood in for her. Then I would switch places and become, also momentarily, mother, father, sister and so on, before then putting a chair, lamp or book in the place of that family member. I have done numerous family sculptures in this manner with only one other person, and while chairs and lamps do not give feedback, one can begin to approximate the family system through using oneself first in those positions. Diagramming on a newsprint easel also helps both client and therapist enormously afterwards. For many clients, enacting their family systems spatially becomes the first time they have had to move from an egocentric position to a multicentric systems position, where they too have to BE each family member in relation to themselves. Such a process suddenly moves them to SEE themselves as part of the whole, also as impacting actors rather than only as receiving victims. Their sense of relationship to themselves and others changes dramatically in this process.

This way of using myself allows me to feel into each person the client is describing. By entering their body postures and gestures for even a brief moment, I can as actress approximate what that person might well be feeling and experiencing in that position and role. This in turn feeds my imagery of what was happening for each person and how that manifested itself interactionally as a total system. Feeding my curiosity, this technique offers me new questions, while giving me an immediate and intimate sense of the interactional context. I can then intervene systemically based on my understanding of the client's images of roles and processes in that interactional context.

ROPE AS METAPHOR FOR "BETWEENNESS"

In another manner of using myself physically, particularly if working with one person, I will use a piece of rope to stand for the dynamic tension of a relationship, with me tugging one end of the rope. When I work with a couple or family, I have them pull on the rope in many different "set-ups" as physical metaphor for ways of relating, for the "betweenness" quality of relationship. In addition to being novel and beyond language, information revealed is simultaneous and experienced. Family members cannot "hide" as they often do in verbal interchange.

When a client is alone and discussing a relationship that he is considering ending, I will toss a short length of rope to him, and ask him to pull on it. Then all of a sudden, I let go. He reacts, and we investigate that reaction: how it felt, what he thought, and the meaning of being "left holding the rope." I then pick up the end of the rope and ask him to pull again, and tell him that at a moment of his own choosing, he will let go of the rope. This is often a startling moment for the client. We then do this and talk about this process, where he is the "leaver" and the rope is metaphor for the relationship between him and his girlfriend. Such active physical concretizations of being the "leaver" or the "leavee" allow meanings and feelings to surface rapidly and for the client to get in touch with many hidden meanings of power/powerlessness involved in ending a relationship, which have prohibited action. The covert is now overt and options and possibilities for new behavior begin to take shape from a different stance.

Relationships have energy and tension in them, which I find that words do not convey very well. The idiosyncratic meanings of relationship words have many nuances. They are "empty-vessel" words, which we each fill with our own images, feelings and meanings. I find that physically concretizing each client's sense of the dynamic tension of a relationship not only fits our earliest way of learning through sensory-motor activity (Piaget, 1952, 1977), but also is a very rapid way to communicate (Duhl,

Kantor, & Duhl, 1973; Duhl, 1983). People easily make their meanings clear for themselves as well as for the therapist. The groundwork is now laid for appropriate interventions on the part of the therapist and for new actions accompanied by new attitudes on the part of the client.

In being free to use myself physically as a vehicle for this type of concretization, I participate in creating metaphors and analogues for clients' real life experience to which we can then refer in quick shorthand. In this process of making meaning overt, I will use myself, my stories, ropes, puppets, wands, toys, drawings and any other object or process, actual or metaphorical, that will create and carry the message. When these types of processes are used with couples and families, all are experiencing something new in that moment, rather than relying on memories and inner images and idiosyncratic word usage. Such active usage of self on the part of the therapist gives family members an alive sense that they too can use themselves in new ways. When people CAN use themselves in new ways, they grow different edges of themselves and in that process create new ways of relating to themselves and in that process create new ways of relating to themselves and others. And that, for me, is what the dance of life and the tasks of therapy are all about.

REFERENCES

Andolfi, M., Angelo, C., Menghi, P., & Nicolo-Corigliano. A.M. (1983). Behind the Family Mask. New York: Brunner/Mazel.

Anonymous. (1972). "Towards the Differentiation of a Self in One's Own Family," in J.L. Framo (Ed.), Family Interaction. A Dialogue Between Family Researchers and Family Therapists. New York: Springer Publishing Co.

Bateson, G. (1979). Mind and Nature. New York: E.P. Dutton.

Bowen, M. (1978). Family Therapy in Clinical Practice. New York: Jason Aronson.

Duhl, B.S. (1976). "The Vulnerability Contract: A Tool for Turning Alienation into Connection in Individuals, Couples and Families." Paper presented at the First International Family Encounter, Mexico City, November 1976.

Duhl, B.S. (1983). From the Inside Out and Other Metaphors. Creative and Integrative Approaches to Training in Systems Thinking. New York: Brunner/Mazel.

Duhl, B.S. (1986). "Toward Cognitive-Behavioral Integration in Training Systems Therapists: An Interactive Approach to Training in Generic Systems Thinking". Journal of Psychotherapy and the Family, Volume I , Number 4, Winter 1985/86.

Duhl, B.S. & Duhl, F.J. (1974). "Another Way of Training Therapists." Paper presented at Nathan Ackerman Memorial Conference of Family Process, Cumana, Venezuela, February 1974.

Duhl, B.S. & Duhl, F.J. (1975). "Cognitive Style and Marital Process." Paper presented at the Annual Meeting of the American Psychiatric Association, Anaheim, CA. May 1975.

Duhl, B.S. & Duhl, F.J. (1981). "Integrative Family Therapy," in A. Gurman and D. Kniskern (Eds.). The Handbook of Family Therapy. New York: Brunner/Mazel.

Duhl, F.J. & Duhl, B.S. (1979). "Structured Spontaneity: The Thoughtful Art of Integrative Family Therapy at BFI". Journal of Marriage and Family Therapy, 1979, 5:3.

Duhl, F.J., Kantor, D., & Duhl, B.S. (1973). "Learning, Space and Action in Family Therapy: A Primer of Sculpture," in D. Bloch (Ed.). Techniques of Family Psychotherapy. New York: Grune and Stratton.

Gordon, W.J.J. & Poze, T. (1973). The Metaphorical Way of Learning and Knowing. 2nd Ed. Cambridge, MA: Porpoise Books.

Minuchin, S. (1974). Families and Family Therapy. Cambridge, MA: Harvard University Press.
Piaget, J. (1952). The Origins of Intelligence in Children. New York: International Universities Press.
Piaget, J. (1977). The Essential Piaget. H.E. Gruber and J.J. Voneche (Eds.). New York: Basic Books.
Satir, V. (1964). Conjoint Family Therapy. Palo Alto: Science and Behavior Books.
Satir, V. (1972a). Speech given at Uses of the Self Conference, New York Family Institute, Southbridge, MA, March 1972.
Satir, V. (1972b). People-Making. Palo Alto: Science and Behavior Books.
von Bertalanffy, L. (1968). General Systems Theory. New York: George Braziller.
Watzlawick, P., Beavin, J.H., & Jackson, D.D. (1967). Pragmatics of Human Communication. New York: W.W. Norton & Co.
Watzlawick, P., Weakland, J., & Fisch, R. (1974). Change. New York: W.W. Norton & Co.

The Person and Practice
of the Therapist:
Treatment and Training

Harry J. Aponte
Joan E. Winter

ABSTRACT. Therapeutic excellence is rooted in a clinician's mastery of both the *technical* and *personal* aspects of treatment. An exploration of the catalytic force of therapy and how it effects the person of the therapist and his use of self generates a number of training implications. A clinical training model, developed at the Family Institute of Virginia, focusing on *the Person and Practice of the Therapist*, is predicated on the assumption that a therapist is most effective when he uses himself for the mutual advancement of both his clients and himself. The model utilizes the various contexts of a therapist's life, including his clinical, collegial, and familial relationships. An excerpted transcript from a training session illustrates a segment of this process.

Clinical training is an intensive learning process undertaken in order to develop the professional skills and competence of a practitioner. It is the bridge that enables and enhances the application of academic and theoretical treatment concepts to the specific clinician within the context of actual therapy. Within the field of psychotherapy, a plethora of models and beliefs about human behavior and change exist. Likewise, an abundance of training interventions and strategies have been developed.

There is one element, however, common to every training model: therapy is conducted by people. In addition, the vehicle for therapeutic change is a social relationship. Consequently, at bottom, the only instrument each training model actually possesses is the "person" of the therapist in a relationship with a client. Despite one-way mirrors, personal psychoanalysis, videotapes, supervision, etc., it is a human person who is alone in a room with a client or a family. In the psychotherapy session, the individual therapist utilizes his expertise and knowledge, as well as his personal life experiences and value system in order to engage with clients in ways that will improve the quality of the clients' lives.

Harry J. Aponte, M.S.W., is Director, The Family Therapy Training Program of Philadelphia, Academy House, # 32D, 1420 Locust Street, Philadelphia, PA 19102.

Joan E. Winter, L.C.S.W., is Director, Family Institute of Virginia, 2910 Monument Avenue, Richmond, VA 23221.

As a result, an intriguing question emerges and challenges the psychotherapy profession: how to develop the competency of the "person of the therapist?" This puzzle is amplified by the trainer's need to simultaneously help the therapist enhance his clinical skills in tandem with his personal skills.

FUNDAMENTAL THERAPEUTIC SKILLS

"*The Person and Practice of the Therapist*" training model emphasizes four essential skills a clinician needs to attain in order to effect a positive therapeutic outcome (Winter, 1982). The areas of expertise include: (1) *external skills*, or the actual, technical behavior utilized by the therapist in the conduct of therapy: (2) *internal skills*, or the personal integration of the therapist's own experiences and self in order to become a useful therapeutic instrument; (3) *theoretical skills*, or the acquisition of theoretical models and conceptual frameworks necessary to identify and guide the therapeutic process; and (4) *collaborative skills*, or the ability to coordinate one's therapeutic efforts with other professionals and agencies, including schools, lawyers, therapists, supervisors, ministers, physicians, or any "significant other" service provider.

Given the differences in treatment methodologies, practically every school of therapy accepts the importance of *theoretical skills*. In most psychotherapy training programs, prior to providing services, it is essential for a practitioner to master a cognitive framework regarding the nature of change for individuals, and frequently for systems. In addition, some training programs note the value of *collaborative skills*, a time honored professional ethic. Despite the fact that, in reality, few models devote training time to the nuts and bolts of developing a practitioner's collaborative abilities, general agreement prevails as to the worth of such skills. Essentially there are two main areas of collaborative skills: (1) with agencies and professionals who provide services other than therapy, and (2) with other psychotherapists.

Due to the complexity of issues facing families today, it is crucial that a therapist understand his own limits, know how to appropriately refer and work effectively with other professionals. The necessity of collaborative skill development is currently heightened by both the increased mobility and technology of today's world and the effect divorce is having on family life (cases requiring collaboration include legal issues such as divorce and child custody, chemical addiction, medical problems, and psychopharmacology, etc.). The opportunity to be the only service provider in today's world is lessening for psychotherapists. Successful clinicians learn how to deal with a variety of contexts and service providers in the client's world. In a family therapy outcome study, Satir kept 96 percent

(57 out of 59) high risk drop-out families engaged in treatment in large measure due to the collaborative approach she utilized with agencies and the court system (Winter, 1986).

The second type of collaborative relationship skills are called for in instances where concurrent treatment is provided by more than one therapist to a family unit. Although outcome research evaluating the effectiveness of two or more therapists concurrently providing service to one family does not indicate change (Gurman & Kniskern, 1981), frequently therapists have little choice but to work concurrently. This is particularly true in divorced and blended family systems, especially if the natural parents do not live in the same locality. Consequently, there is a necessity to master collaborative therapeutic relationships.

Although both *theoretical* and *collaborative* skills are generally viewed as requisite expertise for the clinical practitioner, a major division exists regarding emphasis in teaching technical and personal skills to clinicians. This is especially the case among family therapy training models. Historically, in the field of family, marital or systems therapy, there have been essentially two schools of thought with regard to training. One method focuses on the *external* or the technical and behavioral skills of the therapist, and the other stresses the *internal* skills or the personal integration of the clinician.

Proponents emphasizing external, technical skills (such as Haley and Minuchin[1]) declare that the trainer/supervisor should focus on the actual therapy behaviors displayed by the practitioner and help him acquire the necessary therapeutic respones. For advocates of this method, the practitioner's life is not the object of change or discussion in training. Jay Haley advocates that training for family therapists should be confined to evaluating the metaphor and function of the family's symptom (Minuchin, 1984), and then developing or helping the therapist devise an intervention strategy. Haley asserted that therapists' problems and personal life were not appropriate to the teaching context (Winter, 1986). Specifically, Haley reported that,

> A bill of rights being drafted by clinical students is now in the planning stage. The list includes an item that says no teacher may inquire into the personal life of a therapy student, no matter how benevolently, unless (1) he can justify how this information is relevant to the immediate therapy task in a case, and (2) he can state specifically

---

[1]Recent statements by Minuchin, however, reveal that he has altered his original teaching emphasis on technical skills. He noted,

Many family therapists today are versed in techniques but don't understand families. Sometimes I see marvelous interventions that are incorrect because they are not related to a basic understanding of the family in a social context, but only to the therapist's repertory of interventions. (1984:68)

how this inquiry will change the therapist's behavior in the way desired. (1976:176)

In the externally focused training model, students are given client families and a supervisor. It becomes the job of the supervisor to interpret the meaning and theoretical implications of the client's symptoms and, then, to develop through the trainee's conduct of therapy, an effective technical intervention to alleviate the client's problems.

On the other hand, proponents (such as Bowen and Satir) stressing internal, personal skills hold that the basic task of the training program should be to help the therapist resolve personal conflicts and free himself from his own problems and blind spots. This viewpoint asserts that by assisting the therapist to become more personally integrated, the clinician will be able to intervene with a greater range of choice, insight and creativity in the lives of his clients.

Satir and Baldwin emphasized this perspective:

> The therapist's ability to check on his own internal manifestations is one of the most important therapeutic tools he has. If his internal experience of an interview is different from all other data he is observing and he is fairly sure his reaction is not related to something going on in his personal life, then the most effective way to proceed is on the basis of that internal data. It takes time for the therapist to become aware and be able to trust his internal manifestations, but when he does, he will always have another way to proceed in a therapy situation when he feels stuck. (1983:233)

Murray Brown has taken an unequivocal position about training therapists. Bowen stated, "I am not training people to utilize techniques or telling them how to say hello" (Winter, 1986:302). Bowen realizes that training the person of the therapist should be oriented toward developing an intact, complete person.

The internal, personal skills school of training postulates that when a therapist has resolved his salient problems, he will be cured of some of his selective psychological blindness and will be better able to understand his own psyche and that of his clients. Such a practitioner, it is asserted, has increased access to his own wisdom which enables him to help clients.

Because educational models differ in their focus on skill development and curriculum, trainees are often faced with making an "either-or" choice: to develop expertise in technical or in personal skills. Few clinical programs offer the opportunity to have both supervised treatment with client families, as well as an indepth focus on the practitioner's personal functioning, and how it relates to his conduct of therapy.

Fewer still adopt a flexible training approach that simultaneously integrates the therapist's technical and personal skills. It is uncommon to find a training model that consistently maintains a focus on both the conduct of therapy, with specific case interventions, as well as the therapist's personal issues and the interaction between the two. Systemic links and the interdependence between the therapist and client are frequently overlooked. Specifically, assisting a therapist to incorporate his personal qualities into technical interventions with clients is the core process in the use of self in therapy.

In essence, a person needs both a biological father and mother in order to be born. He needs both a right and left brain in order to make sense out of his world. A therapist needs a training process that can effectively focus on both sides of himself, his technical and personal competence, and that helps integrate the two. Clearly, one can manage with less, but the loss of one or the other dimension, and the lack of amalgamation of the two, will inhibit the range of skills and, consequently, the clinician's effectiveness.

The training approach presented herein, the *Person and Practice of the Therapist (Person-Practice)* model, is the result of two clinicians and teachers, with distinct treatment, training and research experience in both external and internal approaches to training, developing a training system which encompassed both trainers' theoretical models. One trainer's background was primarily Structural family therapy and psychoanalysis. The other trainer had worked indepth with Erickson, Satir and Bowen. Out of this theoretical diversity, and the fact that they jointly devoted four days a month to teaching clinical seminars, a different training process emerged. The *Person/Practice* model is an atheoretical model for training. Very different treatment approaches can be utilized in this training method. Outcome research has revealed, according to Gurman and Kniskern, that selective choice of treatment methodology with specific therapists is a critical variable for change. They asserted,

> The well-worn, but still salient reminder that the ultimate empirical *and* clinical question is, "What treatment for what problem? (with what therapists, etc. etc.) . . . " (1981:748)

Participants in the *Person/Practice* model utilize a variety of treatment strategies in both case discussions and live family interventions, including Structural family therapy, Bowenian family therapy, Satirian family therapy, hypnosis, and organizational development. This training approach does not depend on a specific clinical framework. It utilizes a generic teaching method which can accomodate a variety of technical interventions.

Figure 1 is a paradigm of the four fundamental therapeutic skills underlying the *Person and the Practice of the Therapist* training model. This model holds that each clinician needs expertise, ease and integration in all four dimensions.

Figure 1.

**Four Fundamental Therapeutic Skills:
A Systemic Paradigm**

External   Internal

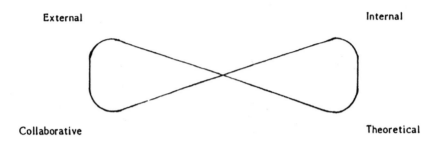

Collaborative   Theoretical

The Figure 8 represents the dynamic movement
inherent in a therapist's emphasis and choice
regarding his skill development.

THEORETICAL FRAMEWORK

Although there are a variety of treatment approaches utilized by the participants training in the *Person/Practice* model, there is a primary value system and theoretical framework that underpins both the treatment and consequent training process. This cognitive map, as noted, does not prescribe a specific treatment intervention strategy for every case or participant. Rather, the theoretical framework is designed to elicit each participant's development of his own beliefs and theory, technical and collaborative skills, and how he uses himself as a person to attain positive outcomes for his clients.

The internal or personal skills of the therapist and its impact on his practice has been an area of inquiry since the inception of psychotherapy. The interaction between the process of therapy and its participation provides definition for training the person of the therapist.

The Person of the Therapist: An Historical Perspective

Not surprisingly, psychoanalysis was the first of the therapies to formally include in its training method a process of understanding and changing the person of the therapist. It was also the first treatment model to emphasize and utilize the relationship between the patient and the therapist as the primary vehicle for ameliorating psychological problems.

Psychoanalysis formally instituted the "training analysis" for the therapist. This model was concerned with the issues inherent in the therapeutic relationship and developed the term transference (for the patient) and counter-transference (for the analyst) to describe their interaction. Freud initially wrote,

> We have become aware of the "counter-transference" which arises in him (the analyst) as a result of the patient's influence on his unconscious feelings, and we are almost inclined to insist that he shall recognize this counter-transference in himself and overcome it . . . . We have noticed that no psycho-analyst goes further than his own complexes and internal resistance permit; and we consequently require that he shall begin his activity with a self-analysis and continually carry it deeper while he is making his observations with his patients. (Freud, 1957:144-145)

Freud believed that the personal reactions of the analyst were critical to the patient's process of change. Counter-transference was viewed by Freud as "unconscious feelings" that were related to the analyst's unresolved, neurotic "complexes." Originally, Freud's solution for counter-transference was self-analysis (which Freud applied only to himself). For his students, he eventually established the training analysis, the precursor of present models of change for the person of the therapist.

Freud worried about "the effect of a constant preoccupation with all the repressed material which struggles for freedom in the human mind . . . stirring up in the analyst . . . all the instinctual demands which he is otherwise able to keep under suppression." He saw the demands of continually facing others' psychological struggles causing problems for the analyst in his own personal and internal life. His concern went so far that he modified his earlier requirement for self analysis to the expectation that the therapist "submit himself to analysis" not once, but "periodically—at intervals of five years or so." In other words, "his own analysis would change from a terminable into an interminable task." Freud was prescribing a continual process of work on self for the analyst (Freud, 1964:249).

Although the *Person-Practice* model espouses the importance of a therapist focusing on and mastering his personal issues in order to function effectively with clients, there are a number of differences from Freud's psychoanalytical approach. First, as indicated, his counter-transference model refers only to the analyst's unconscious "complexes." The *Person-Practice* model draws primarily from the field of systems thinking and family therapy. This theoretical framework incorporates the total life experience of both family and the therapist, conscious and unconscious, real and fantasized. A systems approach holds that "every part is related to the other parts in a way that a change in one brings about a change in all the others. Indeed, everyone and everything impacts and is impacted by every other person, event and thing" (Satir & Baldwin, 1983:191).

The psychoanalytic process, on the other hand, is technically structured to maximize fantasy and projection on the part of the client. The analyst is directed to maintain a passive, almost anonymous position vis-a-vis the patient. In Freud's treatment room, the patient was lying down on a couch, facing a window, with no eye contact, without sitting up and turning his head to see the analyst. Likewise, Freud's chair was at a 90 degree angle to the patient. His view was of an ornate collection of anthropological artifacts.

Contrary to this method, in family therapy the clinician not only sits within the family circle, he plays an active role in creating family change. Outcome studies of family therapy reveal that a therapist's relationship skills (even in behavioral models), elevated activity level, and ability to structure early interviews were related to successful outcome (Gurman & Kniskern, 1981). Whittaker and Keith succinctly concluded, "We are very active as therapists" (1981:207).

Active therapist involvement does not encourage the projective process of transference (which emphasizes the importance of the therapist providing a blank screen or tabula rasa for the patient). Conversely,

> Family therapy requires a use of self. A family therapist cannot observe and probe from without. He must be a part of a system of interdependent people. (Minuchin & Fishman, 1982:2)

Such involvement anchors and increases the reality of transactions between the patient and the therapist. Nonetheless, it is inevitable that both patient and therapist will bring into the therapeutic relationship each person's real and psychological linkages with their respective lives which bear all the scars of their past along with the wounds inflicted by their current lives.

Moreover, from another dimension, because the family therapist plays an active role in the therapeutic relationship, he is less protected than was the analyst from imposing his own personal values and life issues on the patient, especially if the patient's difficulties resonate with those of the therapist (Aponte, 1985). The role of the family therapist demands enormous personal self knowledge and discipline from the practitioner, thus the special necessity of personal work for the family therapist.

 From this perspective, a therapist has a dual clinical task: first, he needs to seek to resolve personal issues that affect his work; and second, learn to recognize and mold who he is, including his flaws, since there is no possibility (as Freud implicitly admitted) that he will ever achieve full resolution of current or past afflictions (Aponte, 1982).

Beyond the historical exploration of this issue, other salient aspects of the therapeutic relationship further clarify the connection between the clinician and his treatment.

Mutuality and Metamorphosis: Implications for the Therapeutic Relationship

In therapy, clients and therapists join together to create a new, actively evolving entity. Each participant brings into therapy his or her distinctive life experiences, world views and personal relationships. In turn, the therapeutic relationship generates yet another set of life experiences. The clinical relationship impacts upon the lives of family members and network associates, even if they are not actual participants in the treatment process. Since the treatment is for the benefit of the client family members, therapeutic transactions are directed by the clinician toward achieving change in the family's life. In the *Person-Practice* model, however, that does not mean that the therapist is inaccessible to being influenced and changed by the family. Indeed, therapeutic affiliations can and do effect the lives of therapists. Each participant in the process takes back to his personal life, to a greater or lesser degree, effects from the therapeutic association.

Therapy is a personal relationship operating within the parameters of a professional structure. Essentially, that professional structure prescribes that the therapist and clients be engaged in their efforts for the beneficial outcome of the family. However, due to the interrelatedness of the participants, a treatment relationship cannot deny the therapist's personal needs. While effective therapy subordinates the therapist's needs to the family's, ideally, the family and therapist should be able to work together in a way that serves and enhances the therapist through the same efforts that are directed toward the family's advancement.

From this perspective, therapists can and should actively conduct treatment in a manner that utilizes all that the therapist is as a person. Learning how to effectively employ the therapeutic alliance in such a comprehensive manner is training the person of the therapist. Within the *Person/Practice* framework, the practitioner must be conscious of what he brings into the relationship and learn to manage himself and his personal dynamics for the welfare of the clients.

Moreover, a clinician needs to be aware of how the therapy he conducts affects him personally. How a person is in the therapeutic relationship should be congruent with the meaning of his own life and his values so that it supports and, perhaps, even contributes to the effort he is making to enhance his own life. Learning to make the therapy he conducts with families work for himself is also part of the training the person of the therapist. These dynamics are crucial forces influencing a clinician's performance and must be addressed in the training of the therapist.

As indicated, the positive outcome of treatment is dependent on the therapist's ability to harness himself within the social relationship of therapy. Successful clinicians learn to be aware of what material they currently bring into the therapeutic process, both strengths and problems, and how to employ these resources for the client's growth and change. Because of the intrinsic interdependence of the treatment process, a practitioner may or may not want to change his personal life in order to better serve the families he treats. Regardless of the therapist's choice in this matter, when his individual issues become an impediment to the client's development, and he is aware of the situation, a sense of discomfort develops. Getting help in problem resolution and management of himself is also training the person of the therapist.

One important side effect resulting from a training focus on the use of self with clients is the reality that, through this process of personal development, the practitioner maintains a greater degree of involvement with his clients and profession. Certainly, this endeavor reduces the prospect of burnout and also increases the therapist's commitment to his clients and to the attainment of a successful therapeutic outcome.

Therapy as a Catalyst for Practitioner Change

Engaging in therapeutic work with clients is a social context which, for a therapist, jostles his own personal issues in ways that few other encounters do. As Freud foretold, the continuous reflection on people's personal struggles leaves little of the therapist's own internal life untouched. Repeatedly, such a process moves a therapist to seek to resolve his own life issues, especially as his dilemmas are inevitably brought to the foreground by the people he is seeing.

From the vantage point of the *Person-Practice* model, training for the person of the therapist becomes an occasion for a clinician to obtain an intervention for himself in the context of his work. Accordingly, as therapists seek to improve their clinical effectiveness, they can also improve themselves.

There are aspects of the person of the therapist that are specifically, and often only, revealed to the clinician through his conduct of therapy. Furthermore, he is not locked into the same person-specific struggles in his work that he has with his own family. He is often more able to pursue change in his work context than at home or in his own personal therapy or analysis. As a consequence, *providing treatment* acts as a potent stimulus to personal growth and fosters a variety of possibilities for change in the therapist himself. This catalyst is rooted in several components of the therapeutic process, including:

Role Structure. Due to the nature of therapeutic roles, the clinician acts as a guide and mentor for his clients. In the course of providing such leadership, he is called upon to risk and reveal himself in ways that may not normally surface in his daily life. The professional role gives him emotional protection and support to risk dealing with aspects of clients' lives, without having to expose or directly examine his own.

Motivation. Repeatedly, therapists have demonstrated a willingness to struggle with and master personal neurotic patterns because they are handicapping their effectiveness with clients and, thus, their professional competence. The desire to attain excellence in one's work is a powerful motivator. If the therapist improves his own life, by assisting his client's functioning, the forceful drive towards both professional achievement and self-actualization are served.

Courage. Clients often call forth a sense of determination in the therapist which he is unable to generate just for himself. Within the therapeutic context, a clinician may be willing to face difficult issues for the benefit of his client which he would not confront just for himself or his own family. For the sake of a commitment to the client, a therapist will travel to unknown territories.

Awareness. In the midst of guiding a client through certain events or life stages, a therapist's awareness may be heightened about issues in his own life which, until that point in time, may have been avoided, suppressed, hidden or buried.

Identification. Treatment outcome studies reveal that an essential element of successful therapy is empathy. As a result of the therapist's process of joining with a family he often develops, in some way, an identification with the client (Freud, 1957). When a practitioner moves into the pain in a client's life, in the accepting and hopeful treatment environment he creates for and with the client, he gains access to similar pain in his own life. Thus, due to the indirectness of his therapeutic transactions, he is better able to endure and face his own failure as a result of the treatment he provides.

Vantage Point. Since the foundation of providing treatment is not for the purpose of changing the therapist, the clinician may be less defensive and more able to observe in this environment. From such a unique vantage point, a powerful paradox emerges: while the therapist is one step removed from the phenomena, he is at the same time through his bond with the client, intimately close to it. This contradictory and inconsistent situation creates a potent indirect passageway to the therapist's psyche. His own protective shield or guard is down since he is not the target of change.

Vicarious Change. A therapist may be changing himself, without his own knowledge, by actively instructing and participating in the client's developmental process. Without awareness, a clinician may have effected a complex, difficult problem within himself. The same directions and suggestions a therapist gives a client he simultaneously gives to his own unconscious mind.

Special Relationships. As in the therapist's personal life, certain clinical relationships can be so challenging or congenial, or in other ways reinforcing or provocative, that they provide a clinician with an unusual learning opportunity. Such therapeutic alliances may support steps toward a practitioner's own desired growth.

Due to these compelling catalytic forces, the *conduct* of therapy can create unique, almost unprecedented opportunities for personal change of the therapist. Curiously, the therapist or his family may have previously been defeated in achieving the very same aim. The process of therapy can generate dynamic movement for both the client and the practitioner. In most instances, the key that unlocks a therapist's successful use of himself, for the beneficial outcome of his clients, is effective clinical training and supervision.

TRAINING MODELS FOR THE PERSON OF THE THERAPIST

A variety of methods training the person of the therapist exist. An overview of predominant models, a summary of the *Person-Practice* method, as well as training transcript explore this dimension.

Overview of Predominant Training Methods

Psychoanalysis approached the development of the person of the therapist through the training analysis, which is independent of the therapist's clinical work except to the extent that his conduct of treatment should happen to overflow into his own analysis (Freud, 1958).

With the advent of a systems approach, family therapy models developed a variety of methods for training the person of the therapist. Most of these models have evolved from the internal or personal skills school of therapy training (Bowen, Satir, Whittaker). The external or technical skills school of training (Haley, Minuchin) has emphasized the therapist's technical interventions and to a lesser degree, theory. Interestingly, Minuchin stated,

. . . for the last fifteen years, I have been teaching an alphabet of skills, which is not a theory but a set of techniques for changing people. At this point, I am dissatisfied with my teaching approach. The idea was: "Okay, let's teach an alphabet of skills and everybody will write his own poem in the end." You begin with an alphabet, then you write your own words and eventually you will write your epic. But many, many people get stuck in alphabets. They are illiterate . . . . Nonetheless, they are presenting themselves as family therapists, even though they have not acquired the wisdom one needs to be an effective people changer. So I think it is time to look at our techniques and to begin to think of a theory. (Minuchin, 1980:8)

Here Minuchin acknowledged the limitations of a narrow focus on techniques. However, his approach to teaching "wisdom" now stresses on theory and knowledge acquisition for the therapist. This perspective omits still the person of the therapist and how he utilizes himself as the instrument of change.

Gurman and Kniskern (1981) in their comprehensive review of family therapy outcome assert that therapist relationship skills have increasingly revealed a relationship to treatment outcome. They stated,

A reasonable mastery of technical skills may be sufficient to prevent worsening or to maintain pretreatment functioning in very difficult cases, but more refined relationship skills are necessary to yield truly positive outcomes in marital-family therapy. (p. 751)

Since the external skills models of treatment and training do not focus on the person of the therapist as a point of inquiry and change, an examination of internal models follows.

Although Bowen would perhaps bristle to be grouped with the personal skills school of training (since he has repeatedly emphasized the need for and development of theory), his training approach, nonetheless, has a clear focus on the development of the person of the therapist. In 1960, Bowen was the first family therapist to present his method of training the person of the therapist to other clinicians, using his own family of origin work as an example. He subsequently printed an "anonymous" paper on his work which became a seminal paper in the family therapy training field (Bowen, 1972).

Bowen diverged from his psychoanalytic background when he proposed that "'training' psychotherapy as we have known in the past (for therapists in training) may one day be considered superfluous" (1972: 164). Parallel to the analysts though, he conceived of a therapist's continual process of "differentiation" (or separating, specializing and distinguishing between) from his own family as an essential ingredient in the development of a mature, effective therapist. Bowen believed that, otherwise, therapists were doomed to displace their own unmet needs on the families they treat (Winter, 1986).

Toward this end, Bowen developed a training approach that "coached" the therapist trainee in his work with his own family of origin, in a type of self analysis with a trainer or therapist acting as a coach. Bowen's method prescribes the usefulness of the therapist researching his family of origin, visiting his family's places of residence, including the ancestral home and, most importantly, learning how it directly related to one's own parents and family members. He postulated, "If you can accomplish half of what you want with your family you are doing great . . . . " (Bowen, 1973). According to Bowen, no family will ever scare or intimidate a therapist as much as his own family, so if a therapist masters his anxiety in his own family, then client families will be "easy" (Bowen, 1973).

Virginia Satir may be the figure in family therapy who has made the development of the person of the therapist most central to her training. As she unequivocally stated, "Our approach assumes that the therapist in his person is the chief tool for initiating change" (Bandler, Grinder & Satir, 1976:2). Her training efforts through the Avanta Network provide month long, residential programs for a group of therapists. In this context, Satir utilizes an indepth method of "Family Reconstruction" for trainees. This process involves an intensive enactment of a therapist's own family dynamics which usually takes at least five hours (Nerin, 1985). Satir's method utilizes workshop participants to play roles in the therapist's family and recreates life events and significant interactions which have effected the therapist. She has three primary goals for this intervention, including: (1) reveal to the therapist the source of his "old learnings" or world view; (2) develop in the therapist an awareness of his parents as people (beyond their role as parents); and (3) assist the therapist in developing his own views and definition of himself (Satir & Baldwin, 1983).

In addition to this intervention technique, Satir and her designated leaders also utilize other methods for therapist change including "Parts Parties" which employs a Gestalt therapy approach to personal integration, and therapist family of origin meetings. By utilizing a group context, away from the therapists' ordinary life context, the therapists are more able to focus on their personal development and use of self.

A basic tenet of Satir's intervention model is committed to the development of the therapist. She stated,

> Using oneself as a therapist is an awesome task. To be equal to that task one needs to continue to develop one's humanness and maturity. We are dealing with people's lives. In my mind, learning to be a therapist is not like learning to be a plumber. Plumbers can usually settle for techniques. Therapists need to do more. You don't have to love a pipe to fix it. Whatever techniques, philosophy or school of

family therapy we belong to, whatever we actually do with others has to be funnelled through ourselves as people. (Satir & Baldwin, 1983:227)

The *Person-Practice* model differs from all of the above training approaches in one major respect: it focuses primarily on the *bridge* between the therapist's personal life and his actual conduct of treatment. The model emerges from an ecological framework with the therapist's clinical practice as the central context or setting for training the person of the therapist.

The Person-Practice Model: Change in Context

Systems thinking suggests that efforts to bring about change for a person should not be limited or circumscribed by any one context of his life. (Context is defined as the interrelated conditions in which something exists or occurs, the setting or environment where a phenomenon manifests itself.) Efforts to bring about change in a person's life most often require work in a variety of interrelated contexts. Change in one context may or may not contribute to change in another context. Successful therapeutic strategies require a considered evaluation regarding which contexts or systems to intervene in to maximize the client's change (Duhl & Duhl, 1981). Likewise, an effective clinical training program must utilize a variety of contexts to impact the therapist, including clinical practice, supervisory relationships, marital relationships, nuclear and family of origin, practice setting, collegial relationships and personal therapy.

In essence, the *Person-Practice* model calls for skillful selection of the context for intervention. The support and development of links between the various contexts enhances the trainee both as a therapist and as a person. The model corresponds to a therapeutic approach which holds that,

Underlying the thinking behind this therapeutic perspective is the assumption that there is a structural continuity between the structural patterns linking the individual, the family and the community, and that an intervention in one of these systems may have a corresponding impact on the others, depending on the strength of the linkages between the organization(s) . . . (Aponte, 1980:332)

GOALS IN TRAINING THE PERSON OF THE THERAPIST

Given an ecological and contextual model for change, the aim of the *Person-Practice* training model is twofold. First, the primary or core purpose of the training is to improve and enhance the quality and success of the therapist's clinical work. Second, a *complementary* goal is to assist the therapist in his efforts toward personal development.

Toward the *primary* goal of enlarging a clinician's therapeutic results: the fundamental treatment objective is to enhance the client's functioning and quality of life. By gaining more understanding and mastery of himself, the therapist does, indeed, gain greater ability to penetrate the meaning of his clients' struggles. Thus, the practitioner effectively utilizes his personal assets and life experiences in the implementation of his technical interventions. When a therapist is not absorbed in his own ego or life situation, he is substantially more able to devote observation skills and energy toward the client. The practitioner's resolution of personal issues not only decreases his projection process, it also allows him to use more of himself with the client and, therefore, increases avenues of change in the therapeutic process.

Toward the *complementary* goal of developing the therapist's own integration: by employing a work related context, which has influential and catalytic forces, training becomes a powerful supplement to the clinician's efforts to move his own life toward greater fulfillment. Training that utilizes and explores with the practitioner the personal context of therapy, and his use of self, becomes an opportunity to invest more in his work and in the people he is treating. The alterations he makes in his life, especially those occasioned by his work, enhance a practitioner's ability to be instrumental in the client's change.

This model implies that a clinician's effectiveness is not limited so much by what he has resolved for himself, but by what he has learned to recognize and work with in himself. Being able to handle certain issues may require in some instances that a clinician achieve a degree of resolution in his personal life, but in *all* circumstances it will mean knowing how to manage within the therapy his reactions to unresolved personal issues in ways that will benefit the client. The point of focus then becomes the context of the therapeutic relationship.

Training and supervision ideally should be designed to help not only a specific case, but also to create an autonomous and effective therapist with all cases. By resolving individual issues, or by learning to work with unchangeable or unresolved issues, a clinician attains greater freedom and ability in his use of self with clients. Moreover, by learning how to relate and manage his personal self, the clinician increases his technical expertise. These goals illustrate the need for an interactive and flexible approach toward therapist development.

PERSON-PRACTICE TRAINING FORMAT

The *Person and Practice of the Therapist* model of training has been formalized at the Family Institute of Virginia in Richmond into a year-long program. The number of trainees in a group is no more than fourteen, and the participants meet monthly for two intensive, consecutive days. In order to acquire sufficient clinical skills, most people participate for at least two years. On a rotating basis, each trainee has an individual presentation time, designed to examine a clinical or personal dilemma, or conduct a live family interview. Prior to making the presentation, the trainee prepares a written description for class distribution analyzing his selected issue. The written assessment is intended to help develop the therapist's theoretical and conceptual skills. Additionally, it intensifies his personal involvement and understanding of the selected issue.

A trainee presents to two leaders, male and female, and to their colleagues in the group who act as a source of support, feedback and challenge. The training program gives each participant a variety of contexts where he may address individual issues as they relate to his personal life and clinical performance.

Presentation formats each have a different merit, and therapists are encouraged to make use of methods, including:

Discussion of Personal or Clinical Issues. In this medium, a therapist presents a clinical case or personal issue to the leaders. He utilizes the transactions between himself, the leaders and group members, to better understand the case, himself, and the interaction between the two. Additionally, he explores consequent clinical strategies.

Videotape or Audiotape of a Clinical Session or Training Presentation. Such recordings provide a possibility to observe the therapist in action. This method affords an opportunity to focus on and analyze a treatment segment of any length. It allows the clinician the prerogative to see himself and get clinical suggestions. In this method, he can also view both the clinical and training tape by himself when the group is over.

Role Play of a Clinical Issue. The leaders have a chance, with the direct involvement of group members, to make observations and intervene with a therapist in vivo. This simulation provides safety and the freedom to experiment not offered in a live or videotaped therapy session. Therapist and role-playing clients are asked to spontaneously create a treatment situation or problem. Such enactments draw from the participants fresh reactions to each other, and allow for the possibility of a "take two," corrected intervention.

Live Session With Patient Family or Own Family. The live session provides the most direct opportunity for the leaders to intervene with a therapist around his clinical work or personal life. In interviews with a therapist's own family, the therapist and leaders pursue identified issues with usually one of the leaders conducting the session, while the other leader and the group view through an observation mirror. In interviews with patient families, the leaders can observe from outside the interview room, telephone input to the therapist, or can join the therapist with his clients.

An important element of this clinical training method is the utilization of videotape. Each therapist's presentation is taped to permit review on his own time. He can do this alone, with other group participants, his own family members, personal therapist or other professional colleagues. Once more, this creates a linkage between the various contexts in his life. When a live clinical interview is taped, the therapist can review it with the clients. In this context, the person has the opportunity to hear and see what he did not before. Participants can share with others who are not part of the training group and experience the presentation in yet another context. Each trainee has an individual six-hour tape, which he can review at the end of the year and evaluate his progress.

In the course of a year, a therapist's decision to focus on his personal life or his therapy shifts. Regardless of whether the principal concern at a point in time is his clinical work or his personal life, he is expected to examine both arenas during the training program. In the *Person-Practice* training method, each participant selects a concentration for his professional growth and change. At various times a therapist will be motivated to acquire skills in different dimensions. The clinical program remains adaptable in order to accomodate the trainees' individual differences. The pattern of a person's life is inextricably woven into his choice of skill concentration. The variability each trainee exercises, coupled with the format's flexibility, provides a variety of experiental opportunities for the trainees.

Occasionally, a trainee only feels comfortable presenting in one dimension. For example, some therapists may feel safer presenting a case from a strictly clinical viewpoint, or vice versa, some therapists are afraid to reveal their practice skills and enjoy talking about themselves. Since the model holds that *internal* and *external* skills as well as *theoretical* and *collaborative* expertise are instrumental in creating competent practitioners, a trainee may need to be encouraged to look at and risk himself in another dimension. There may be strategic reasons for encouraging a therapist to work on one area at a moment in time. Once safety and trust have been established between the leaders and the group, however, shifts in skill emphasis usually occur. At the beginning of training, the leaders often need to guide the trainees in the choice of skill development. However, as a therapist develops personal and clinical mastery, his choice of emphasis tends to be more congruent with his needs.

The following transcript illustrates the range and variability of both external and internal skill development in one participant. Included is a transcript of a training session and the trainee's written reaction to that intervention. Finally, a transcript of a live therapy interview the trainee conducted, with the leaders' supervision, at the following training seminar one month later. Several contexts, including clinical practice, case evaluation, marital relationship, family of origin dynamics, personal therapy, colleagueal relationships, and practice setting are exemplified.

TRANSCRIPTS FROM A TRAINEE'S PRESENTATION

A trainee, Devan, presented a clinical problem for discussion. She wanted a case consultation because she knew she was having an unusual amount of difficulty in helping a couple she was treating. She presented the case to the two leaders, J and H, in the group's presence. The entire intervention took approximately one hour. The excerpted transcript begins when Devan is revealing how the wife had recently stopped an affair.

> D: . . . the event that got her to stop the affair . . . I mean the therapy event that four weeks ago, she came in and told me . . . and told me that she had talked to this daughter about the affair, and I just went crazy. And I told her that that was awful . . .
> H: She was trying to get her daughter to collude with her?
> D: Yeah, and I just really told her that that was just unacceptable and that I was no longer willing to have that information and have her daughter know and we know, and her know, and her husband not know, and that she either had to cut it off completely and stop it, as in *now*, or I was going to make her deal with her husband about it. I was really upset with her and uncomfortable about the three women having the secret and her continuing to be duplicitous and then dumping that on the daughter. But, it was clear that it took her daughter for me to get that clear about it, you know it took her . . . (inaudible) . . daughter for me to decide.
> H: That's what I was going to ask you . . . it has been quite a while . . . to have this kind of secret . . .
> D: Right, and I have been saying all along, "stop it, stop it," but I have never just actually thrown a fit and said I am not going to collude with you any more until she used her daughter.

Devan started by describing that she had strong personal convictions that it was wrong for the woman to maintain this deception with her husband, and to attempt to involve the therapist in maintaining the secret. Devan could not, however, take a decisive position with the woman until the information surfaced that the daughter had subsequently become involved in the secret. The co-leader, underlined her struggle by his questioning. A short time later in the presentation, Devan identified a personal reason why this case was difficult for her.

H: . . . sort of brought allusions to your marriage, a hint that there
is some connection between your marriage and this marriage.
D: (My husband) and I had this discussion about a week
ago . . . the reason why I decided to present this is because we are
having this discussion about a week ago. I wasn't understanding
what he was saying, and he said, "If you had a client that was like
this and was saying this to you, what would you do?" I said, "Actually, I do have a client. And I don't know what to do with them." I
am stuck with them.
H: I see.
D: So, the connection is real clear to me. In this particular couple
that connection is clear to me. I have two other couples that I also
really don't feel really like I am doing dynamite therapy with, and
their specific issues are not as clear to me. With them (all three
cases) the generic issue is that the men are not very expressive, kind
of withdrawn, deny that there are problems, say that it is their
wives' problems that there is a marriage, that there is a depression,
and that they want me to fix their wives . . . that one of them drinks
too much and doesn't think he has a drinking problem, and in both
of those other two couples . . . also I feel as if when I meet with the
men individually I can connect with them and I can say . . . you
know, I can be real direct with them and it feels okay. When I get
there with a couple, I feel like I am not absolutely doing anything
and at the end of the couple's session, my impulse is to take the wife
and say, "Get a good lawyer."

H: Right, you identify with the woman and distance yourself from
the men.
J: And it says here (in Devan's case presentation commentary written before the seminar). "Maybe she should go get her happiness
where she can." Does that say anything to you?

D: Yeah, as a matter of fact, I thought about whiting out that sentence, but then . . . I thought . . . no, I would go ahead and do it.
That is why I am here. Well, I am real clear that I can identify in
here, not only her and me, but I can also identify her and my mother . . . about wanting this man to give her something. She wants
him to say . . . I mean, she just wanted some . . . Anne (the woman) is saying . . . she said to him, "I just need you to tell me that
you love me." Well, she told him that when they got separated in
June, and since June, he hasn't told her that he loves her. He refuses
to tell her that he loves her, he tells her that he likes her okay, he
tells her that he needs her, but he refuses to say the words to her, "I
love you," because she asked him to . . . . So, there is a part of
me, when he starts pulling that chill on her that really feels like

"you don't need this crap." You know. Because I don't think that the things she is asking him for are that far out of . . . are that far out.

The co-leader, J, then further explores Devan's emotional entanglement with the woman.

J: (The other man) moved away from the time she stopped the affair?
D: When she told him that she was absolutely not going to see him any more. But see, all summer she has been going to him and saying, you know . . . you knew she was in therapy and she has been going to him, and saying "we've got to cut this off." He threatened to kill himself if she cut him off. It has just been one of those . . .
J: I don't understand why you see yourself as really identified with . . . her, and involved with her, and all this, when she lies to you like this. I don't understand where you are, you know . . . you are so involved and on her side.
D: Well, because I guess I feel sorry for her. I feel like she is, she is much more clear with her pain.

D: Well, I guess the mental machination that I do in this head is that I see her as not being in control of this. I see her as being helpless and confused, and just not . . .
J: She is entitled to anything that she wants to because her husband doesn't say that she is attractive. She is entitled to mistreat you, mistreat her daughter . . . because he doesn't "mow mow" and "wow wow" over her. Is this . . . I am trying to find out where your vulnerability is.

D: I mean one of the first things that comes to my mind, but I am sure this isn't all of it, one of the first things that comes to my mind, is that she acts much more kind of helpless and depressed, and you know all of her symptoms are like my mother. And so, I am much more able to respond to that and take care of her inspite of what she is doing. The other part that comes to me is that there is like a . . . it is really a shitty thing to be doing to him (the husband) and the second part that comes to me is that I wonder if I am not, if there wasn't some kind of underlying motivation for me about the power that I got from being that shitty to him.

H: The picture I get of you is both contexts: as the wife, as the woman who gets what she can, and as the woman who will seduce the guy but not really give herself to him, is the somebody who doesn't trust anyone, who is basically alone and says, "I have got to have all the strength myself. I can't depend on anyone."

H: But, if you follow this scenario as I pointed it out, and if you (and your husband) were in therapy and he is having the affair, and the male therapist that you were seeing really got you to let down your guard with him, so you cry to him and you came to depend upon seeing him and then found that he has that secret and that he was saying to (your husband), "Why don't you ditch this broad anyway. She's not going to deliver."

D: Whew! I am sitting here feeling real scared and vulnerable because . . . that is really shitty therapy. I am really feeling real vulnerable about that part of me, besides the other part, because it is just like real bad . . . I am wondering how I get myself out of it, dig myself out of the hole.

H: My question is, can you get that scared about what you do to you in your personal life as you get about what you do in your therapy? Are you as guarded in your personal life?

D: I don't feel like I have people who I trust except maybe . . . sometimes alternately, I trust (my husband) and sometimes I don't . . . and I trust my mother, you know . . . that's about it.

D: You see, I don't know if people would even . . . it is like, what is wrong with me is that I don't really know how to be honest with people. I lie a lot. Some of them are just little lies, some of them are bigger. I lie a lot. In order to be close to me, people are going to have to take the time. I am going to have to not lie, you know. I am getting to have to stop playing those games.

H: Are you in therapy?

D: Yeah, but I . . . I don't trust my therapist.

H: Then you're not in therapy. That is the function of your therapist. And, see the thing is, that you are not taking that risk with your therapist.

J: But have you really decided that you are tired of suffering, you are tired of this lonely . . .

D: Oh, yeah. I have had it with . . . I have been tired of it for six weeks. Ever since I had a severe case of the flu. I have been tired of it. I am not going to do . . . I am not going to live like this. I have been trying to do what I know to do, you know . . .

The therapist revealed that she identified with the woman's deception with people because she, like her client, did not trust that people would care for her if they knew her as she knew herself. The presentation also dealt with how much Devan wanted her husband's love and commitment, but how fearful she was of openly testing her marriage, lest her husband fail her. Later, she expressed her desire to surface those issues directly with her husband. Additionally, Devan voiced her determination to deal with her own therapist, whose approval she also wanted and feared losing. Since co-workers were in the group, Devan talked directly with them about her long standing anxiety that they would not want to work with her, nor would they want her friendship. Devan walked out of the presentation indicating a determination to be straightforward with the people in her life. She committed to help Anne, the wife, develop the courage and take the personal risks required to reach out for the love she, too, wanted from her husband.

Subsequent to this intervention, Devan reviewed an audiotape of her previous presentation and reported how listening to the tape affected her. First she addressed the personal effect of the tape on her:

One morning I was here early and had a few hours set aside for administration. The transcript was on top of the pile of papers, so I picked it up and decided to listen to a few pages of the tape. As it turned out, I spent 2 1/2 hours without moving from my chair and finished the tape. It felt like I was in some kind of trance or altered state . . . . I was totally focused on the process of how the presentation was unfolding.

I was also aware that I was processing the tape on at least two levels. The therapist in me was saying, "what an interesting case study," and was focused on the interview skills of H and J, and how they fit together as a co-therapy team. I was struck by how involved they were with "the client" (me) and how direct they were about their sense of what was going on. The "I" part of me went through some of the struggle all over again. I could literally see J's eyes tearing up while she asked me if I believed she would kick me out of the practice; and I felt kind of sad and ashamed that H was *so* right when he accused me of not reaching out to people and then blaming them for my loneliness.

I had the sense of humanness of the whole . . . thing and a feeling of universality. I don't know, just that me, the person, and me, the therapist, are always growing and changing, and so is everyone in that group experience, and so are my clients. And it just felt like a type of circular "watering process." The flowers grow because they are watered, and they produce moisture that goes into the air and forms clouds that water the flowers, etc. Anyway, that was the trance.

Then Devan described the effect listening to the tape had on her clinical work:

I finished the tape on a Wednesday and that afternoon, I had a few families to see, but no noticeable effect from the morning's experience. The next day, though, I did three separate hours of therapy with three women clients that were absolutely different from any therapy I have ever done. It was like watching myself do therapy, almost like I was really in there with these women and I was taking risks with them, and touching them (literally, at one point, I was physically holding on of my clients), and another voice was saying, "Good God," and I was not afraid of myself. I knew (really knew) that my confrontation wouldn't destroy them (or me) and that we were in it together. It's really hard to put into words, but I just felt "on" and exhilarated and gleeful in a way I haven't ever felt as an individual therapist. I have sometimes in the past gotten some of that same feeling with a really difficult family, when I know I'm right at the core of the issue and that the family absolutely will leave the room changed. But never with an individual client. It's always been too risky to get in there with them and possibly lose (myself?), or lose control or whatever. This time I didn't, though, and it was *so* real, and during the past week, I have felt moments like those. They aren't as steady as they were that day, but they are more often and it's somewhat like following a map or playing hide and seek with myself. I have a hint now when I took the right fork in the road or when I'm getting hot or cold. I'm not always choosing to move toward hotter (sometimes I run for the ease and safety of cold), but I know it's there and it's possible.

One month later, in Devan's next presentation in the training group, she conducted a session in which she was supervised live by the leaders. The client Devan interviewed was a different one than in the earlier presentation made to the training seminar, but the themes of trust and honesty were the same. This client was a young woman (twenty-two) who had been having an affair with a married man.

> D: How do you feel about the way things are between us in therapy?
> C: I guess right now they're sort of like at a standstill. I mean, it could go either way. You know, it was like improvement and then, stop, it's just right there.
> D: What do you think that's about?
> C: I don't know, I guess it's just, I don't know. I mean, I've been honest as far as . . . .
> D: You've been honest?
> C: Yeah, with you, as far as what's going on here and at home and at work, you know . . . .
> D: But there are a lot of situations that you and I haven't (sic) gotten into where you were not honest with me.
> C: Um, no, I feel like I've been honest with, well . . . .
> D: I felt like you weren't being honest with me on a couple occasions.
> C: Like, specifically.
> D: Well, content-wise, there have been a couple of situations where you told me a half truth. Like, specifically, the time I tried to

schedule the doctor's appointment for you and you said you couldn't make it because you were meeting friends, and you weren't meeting friends; you were meeting Ray. So I felt like it was not complete, my information was not complete and I was being led to believe you were in one situation when you were in another. I think I've even told you before that I thought you were lying to me . . . .

At this point, Devan was able to face with her client the deficits in their therapeutic relationship. The therapist was aware, unlike her presentation a month before, of the dishonesty in the client and how that trait spilled over into other aspects of her life, including the therapy.

D: I'm saying that's what needs to change. I need to go out on a limb and you need to go out on a limb for us to develop some trust.
C: Well, uh huh.
D: How do you feel about what I'm saying? I feel like I'm saying some pretty difficult things and you have on your pretend person here.
C: I'm just listening, I mean, I don't know what to say . . . I mean, of course, I don't like when I say those things because I know I don't mean them. But I guess when I'm hurting I want someone else to hurt I just make up lies or scare them. It's the only way I know.
D: What do you think would happen if you called me and said, Devan, I'm really hurting and feeling lonely, and I need to talk for a few minutes so I can calm down . . . .
C: Well, that sounds better than what I do now.
D: Do you think I would say "no" and hang up on you unless you're threatening to kill yourself or run away or something?
C: No, but I just remember one day when I made four phone calls to four people in my family to let them know how I was feeling and, yet, they were too busy and didn't have time to talk. All in the same week—to my brother, my sister, my father and mother. And each one said, "I don't have the time," click, "I don't have the time," click.
D: Did you tell them what you needed?
C: No.
D: Well, see, I think that's the key here, because I see that happening with your family, and it probably happens with other relationships. It probably happens between you and me, too. Because if you come in and pretend it's all nice and hunky dory, and never say what you really need then they let you down and they don't ever know how badly they hurt you.

Devan was able to risk engaging with her client in a confrontation over the client's trust of her. She was able to see the client's loneliness and how she protected herself from intimacy, as Devan herself does, for fear of rejection. Additionally, she was able to effectively address the client's affair without becoming personally entangled or threatened by the therapeutic material.

CONCLUSION

Much is expected of therapy. It is the vehicle by which people attempt to change their losses into fulfillment. Therapy has become a modern day tool to address the interaction and complexities between people and their environment. The instrument common to every therapeutic model is the person of the therapist in a relationship with the client. Considering the clinician's task, it is no wonder that the person of the therapist and his use of self become a central focus of inquiry.

The *Person/Practice* model is an atheoretical, generic training approach, not bound to any specific school of therapy. It focuses primarily on the *bridge* between the therapist's personal life and his actual conduct of treatment. The model strives to enhance the psychotherapist's ability to utilize his own life experiences, personal assests and struggles in behalf of his professional performance. The training is aimed toward generating effective therapeutic outcomes and supplementing the clinician's efforts to advance his own life. The learning context is focused on the practitioner's actual conduct of therapy, utilizing live supervision, videotapes and cases or personal presentations within a colleagueal training group.

From the perspective of the *Person/Practice* model, a process that fully explores with a therapist the personal context of his work and how to master himself within that framework is a bedrock element of clinical training. The approach postulates that when a person's work becomes an opportunity to improve himself, he makes a greater commitment to the people he is treating and discovers new avenues to improve the quality of his client's lives. In essence, helping a therapist to utilize his personal qualities in clinical or technical interventions is the core process in the use of self in therapy.

REFERENCES

Aponte, H.J. (1980). Family therapy and the community. In Margaret S. Gibbs, Juliana Rusic Lachenmeyer, and Janet Sigal (Eds.), *Community psychology, theoretical and empirical approaches* (pp. 311-333). New York: Gardner.

Aponte, H.J. (1982, March-April). The person of the therapist, the cornerstone of therapy. *The family therapy networker*, (pp. 19-21, 46).

Aponte, H.J. (1985). The negotiation of values in therapy. *Family Process. 24*, 323-338.

Bandler, R., Grinder J. & Satir, V. (1976). *Changing with families*. Palo Alto, CA: Science and Behavior.

Bowen, M. (1971-1974). *Murray Bowen family therapy seminars.* Seminar presentations at the Medical College of Virginia, Richmond, VA.

Bowen, M. (1972). Toward a differentiation of a self in one's own family. In James L. Framo (Ed.), *Family interaction* (pp. 111-173). New York: Springer.

Duhl, B.S., & Duhl, F.J. (1981). Integrative family therapy. In A.S. Gurman and D.P. Kniskern (Eds.), *Handbook of family therapy* (pp. 483-513). New York: Brunner/Mazel.

Freud, S. (1957). The future prospects of psycho-analytic therapy. In J. Strachey (Ed. and Trans.) *The standard edition of the complete works of Sigmund Freud* (Vol. XI, pp. 144-145). London: Hogarth Press. (Original work published 1910.)

Freud, S. (1958). Papers on technique: Editor's introduction. In J. Strachey (Ed. and Trans.) *The standard edition of the complete psychological works of Sigmund Freud* (Vol. XII, p. 87). London: Hogarth Press.

Freud, S. (1964). Analysis terminable and interminable. In J. Strachey (Ed. and Trans.) *The standard edition of the complete psychological works of Sigmund Freud* (Vol. XXIII, p. 249). London: Hogarth Press. (Original work published 1937.)

Gurman, A.S. & Kniskern, D.P. (1981). Family therapy outcome research: Knowns and unknowns. In A.S. Gurman and D.P. Kniskern (Eds.), *Handbook of family therapy* (pp. 742-775). New York: Brunner/Mazel.

Haley, J. (1976). *Problem solving therapy* (pp. 176-177). San Francisco: Jossey-Bass.

Minuchin, S. (1980, Vol. IV, No. 3). (Interviewed by Richard Simon, Ed.). A therapy of challenge. *Family Therapy Practice Network Newsletter*, (pp. 5-11).

Minuchin, S. & Fishman, C.H. (1982). *Family therapy techniques.* Cambridge, MA: Harvard University Press.

Minuchin, S. (1984, November-December). (Interviewed by Richard Simon, Ed.) Stranger in a strange land. *Family Therapy Newsletter*, (pp. 20-31, 66-68).

Nerin, W.F. (1986). *Family reconstruction: Long day's journey into light.* New York: W. W. Norton.

Satir, V., & Baldwin, M. (1983). *Satir step by step.* Palo Alto, CA: Science and Behavior.

Whitaker, C.A., & Keith, D.V. (1981). Symbolic-experiential family therapy. In A.S. Gurman and D.P. Kniskern (Eds.), *Handbook of family therapy* (pp. 187-225). New York: Brunner/Mazel.

Winter, J.E. (1982). *Philosophy of supervision.* (No. 2511004). Richmond, VA: Commonwealth of Virginia, Board of Behavioral Sciences.

Winter, J.E. (1986). *(Family Research Project: Family Therapy Outcome Study of Bowen, Haley, Satir).* Unpublished 1978-1980 interview transcripts.

The Effective Family Therapist:
Some Old Data and Some New Directions

Alan S. Gurman

ABSTRACT. Although family therapy researchers to date have provided no direct tests of hypotheses related to the therapist's "use of self," some data do exist on the broader, but closely related, question of what constitutes an effective family therapist, in terms of both enduring individual characteristics and styles of behavior in the actual conduct of therapy. This paper reviews existing data on this question, and addresses certain matters pertaining to the impact of research on clinical practice, as considered in the context of the question of what constitutes an effective family therapist.

The matter of what light research might throw on the qualities of the effective psychotherapist is one which has received a great deal of attention in literature of individual psychotherapy (Gurman & Razin, 1977), but very little attention in the literature of family therapy (Gurman & Kniskern, 1978b, 1981). Thus, when I was invited by the College[1] to address the question, "What is an effective family therapist?", the words of Mark Twain came quickly to mind. Twain said, "I was gratified to be able to answer promptly, and I did. I said I didn't know." Indeed, Twain had anticipated by about one century the characterization of researchers suggested recently by Pittman (1981), who wrote:

> Researchers are different from normal people, and particularly different from theorists. Researchers are never quite sure of anything, and the longer they do the research, the less sure they become. The more they doubt, the more they learn. The more they understand, the more they change. The more they reverse themselves, the more they confuse everybody else. Most of the theorists are reformed researchers who gave up their doubt. (p. 5)

It is in this context of uncertainty that I will try to clarify the befuddling

---

Alan S. Gurman, Ph.D., is the Editor of the *Journal of Marital and Family Therapy*, and Professor of Psychiatry, University of Wisconsin Medical School, 600 Highland Avenue, Madison, WI 53792.

[1]This paper is a revised version of the author's keynote address to the Child and Adolescent Psychiatry Section Meeting, Royal College of Psychiatrists, London, England, March 1982.

and unscrew the inscrutable. I would also like to offer some thoughts about ways of addressing the issue of what constitutes an effective family therapist that may be both more useful and compelling to clinicians than those which researchers have used until now. As will be seen, the amount of existing research on this essential question is scant, indeed. One may speculate that the near dearth of research on such matters has been part and parcel of the dominant trends in the field of family therapy toward technique-oriented vs. relationship-oriented models of treatment. Indeed, there probably exist no research data which directly address clinically and theoretically important questions concerning the "use of self" in family therapy. Still, therapist characteristics measured both inside and outside the context of treatment, and repetitive patterns of behavior in treatment certainly constitute very real and important aspects of the person of the family therapist, and thus are of genuine relevance to the topic of this special issue on "The Use of Self" in family therapy.

WHAT DO WE KNOW ABOUT THE EFFECTIVE FAMILY THERAPIST?

Therapist Variables Measured Outside of Therapy

First, we know that this is not the right way to ask the very question we want to answer: we must ask this question in more refined ways, and actually must ask at least two different questions to find our answers: (1) Are there therapist characteristics which affect outcomes, for better or for worse, independent of particular families? (2) What therapist characteristics that are manifest in interaction with families influence therapy outcomes?

Asking the first question assumes, of course, "that those therapist characteristics identified outside of treatment remain stable *and* are manifested in the treatment setting independent of the patient (family)," and that "the effect of the manifested therapist variable under study is constant for all patients (families)" (Parloff, Waskow, & Wolfe, 1978, p. 234).

Five major categories of relevant therapist characteristics measured outside the therapy session have been identified in the past (cf: Gurman & Kniskern, 1978b, 1981; Parloff et al., 1978): the therapist's personality, mental health, experience level, sex, and other demographic variables, such as race and socioeconomic status.

Personality characteristics. Personality characteristics include, among other things, the therapist's attitudes, beliefs and values about intimate relationships, ethnic differences, mental health and pathology, and so on (Rabkin, 1977). To date, there have been no studies of any of these therapist personality characteristics in family therapy.

Relevant enduring personality characteristics also include certain "human" qualities. Parloff et al. (1978) have noted that "The various prescriptions for the ideal psychotherapist have included a litany of virtues more suited perhaps to the most honored biblical figures than to any of their descendents" (p. 235). Although such laudatory therapist characteristics as honesty, perceptiveness, empathy, open-mindedness, caring, and the like would be blasphemous to impugn, there exist few data in the family therapy field to bolster the everyday convictions of therapists that such human qualities make a difference in terms of outcome.

Mental health. A related set of variables, which may be called the "therapist's mental health," have also been touted widely as bearing significantly on the outcomes of psychotherapy. While some influential figures in the family field, such as Haley (1976), have either dismissed the therapist's own mental health as being irrelevant to the effective practice of family therapy, or have simply not addressed the matter explicitly, others argue that the therapist's mental health and psychological integrity are essentially factors in helping families to change. Skynner (1981), for example, has taken the position that "the therapist's psychological health . . . is the most crucial attribute in the therapist . . . he must be at ease with himself, able to enjoy himself, relatively satisfied with his life, his marriage, his sexuality and his family" (p. 75). And, in the Bowenian perspective, it has been asserted that "it is difficult for a family to grow beyond the level of differentiation of its therapist" (Kerr, 1981, p. 256). While such assertions are quite consistent with the models of family health and the models of family change from which they derive, they remain entirely unconfirmed. Indeed, such assertions have never been tested. Nor have assertions about the value of personal therapy of any sort for family therapists been tested.

Sex. Thus far, only one study (Santa-Barbara, 1975; Woodward et al., 1975) of the effect of therapist gender on outcomes has appeared, and it is contaminated and confounded in numerous ways (Gurman & Kniskern, 1978b). While every family therapist probably needs to engage in some sex, there is no evidence that being of one sex or the other has any reliable impact on the effectiveness of family therapy.

Experience level. There is good reason to predict that one might find increased experience as a family therapist being associated with better therapeutic outcomes. While several studies suggest such a relationship (Freeman et al., 1969; Griffin, 1967; Roberts, 1975; Schreiber, 1966; Shellow et al., 1963), and also suggest that more experienced family therapists have lower dropout rates (Gurman & Kniskern, 1978a), the asserted association has been tested quite inadequately. For example, experience as a family therapist has rarely been ascertained separately from experience as a psychotherapist in the more general sense. While many family therapists (e.g., Haley, 1976) argue vehemently that experience as a psychotherapist (usually taken to mean as an individual psychodynamically oriented psychotherapist) is likely to decrease (or even preclude) one's effectiveness in treating families, such a position must be said to have the status only of a proselytizing polemical platitude. And, while others believe that a backlog of experience as an individual therapist enhances the efficacy of family therapists who work in accordance with either psychodynamic principles (e.g., Gurman, 1981; Sager, 1981; Skynner, 1981), or in accordance with, e.g., structural or strategic principles, this view also remain unsupported by data.

An interesting variation on this experience theme involves the evidence which suggests that experience level differences between co-therapists in family therapy may lead to less positive clinical outcomes (Gurman, 1974, 1975; Rice et al., 1972). Such less than optimal outcomes are apparently mediated by the "felt competition" in such co-therapist pairings (Rice et al., 1972).

Demographic variables. Such demographic variables as race (Sattler, 1977), social class (Lorion, 1973) and ethnicity (McGoldrick, Pearce, & Giordano, 1982) presumably exert powerful influences on the interactions between therapists and the families they treat. The stereotypes held by therapists about the families they treat certainly can, and do, at times lead to inadequate treatment. Both the absence of common experiences and the presence of differing values about intimacy and conflict, roles, dealing with the world outside the family etc., as well as ignorance of different rules about such matters in different ethnic groups, may interfere with establishing a working therapeutic alliance. Obviously, such therapist demographic variables can only exert influence for better or for worse in combination and in interaction with analogous family characteristics. Thus far the interactive consequences of similarities and differences on such variables remain untested in family therapy. Moreover, demographic differences such as ethnicity probably do not have universal effects on either the process or outcome of family therapy, but probably vary, in complex fasion, with both the type of presenting problem and the type of therapy.

Therapist Variables Measured in the Process of Therapy

By far, the most consistent findings of relevance to the characterization of the effective family therapist have come from studies of the therapist plying her trade, that is, assessed in the actual conduct of treatment. These in-process variables may be referred to as therapists' "styles" and therapists' relationship skills.

Therapist "styles." The term "style" refers to "the manner or mode of the therapist's expression, independent of the content of such expression" (Parloff et al., 1978). Given the prominence attributed to content-free ways of relating in family therapy generally (Gurman & Kniskern,

1981), it is indeed, disheartening that there has been so little empirical study of the dimensions of therapist style that make a difference in family therapy. Thus far, there is a modicum of evidence that the family therapist's ability to model meaning clarification (Jones, 1969) and positive perceptions of family members (Graham, 1968) are important both for successful engagement in treatment and for ultimate outcome. Some especially important findings, which are entirely consistent with every influential model of family therapy (cf: Gurman & Kniskern, 1981), show that more active family therapists have fewer early dropouts than less active therapists, and that families respond more positively in early sessions to expressions of the therapist's involvement than to expressions of mere understanding (Shapiro, 1974; Shapiro & Budman, 1973). Interestingly, there is evidence that a family therapist's "structuring skills" (directiveness, clarity, self-confidence) also are associated with different degrees of therapeutic improvement (Alexander et al., 1976; Alexander & Parsons, 1973).

Therapeutic "relationship skills." Consistent with findings in virtually every other area of psychotherapy research, the familiar triad of therapist empathy, warmth, and related relationship-building skills, have been found to be salient in research on the outcomes of family therapy (Alexander et al., 1976; Waxenberg, 1973; DeChenne, 1973). It is important to note, however, that such therapist skills have not yet been studied in the practice of most methods of family therapy. Still, there is evidence that at least some minimal level of empathic responsiveness is needed to assure completion of therapeutic tasks in even the most behavioral of family therapies (Gurman & Knisker, 1978b).

The most compelling findings on the power of therapist style and skill variables has been found in the literature on therapist variables which are associated with deterioration, or negative effects, in family therapy. There appears to be a particular therapist manner of relating which increases the changes of negative outcomes. This manner of relating has been described as "one in which the therapist does relatively little structuring and guiding of early treatment session, uses frontal confrontations of highly affective material very early in therapy rather than stimulating interaction, gathering data, or giving support; and does not actively intervene to moderate interpersonal feedback in families in which one member has very low ego-strength" (Gurman & Kniskern, 1978a, p. 11).

If the ideal characteristics to which every family therapist may aspire define the essence of being a therapeutic "mensch," then this description of the deterioration-inducing family therapist must certainly define what can only be called a therapeutic "schlemeil." "Mensches" probably achieve good outcomes in almost any type of psychotherapy, and "schlemeils," poor outcomes. From a different vantage point, it is probably the case that the effective family therapist needs to be both a mensch and a skilled technician, and, most of all, needs to know how and when and with whom to be what. Some families need only genuine nurturance from the therapist; others need the therapist to be an organizational consultant, and still others may need the therapeutic experience to be something of an educational seminar. Shifting one's way of relating from family to family is not ingenuine; indeed, it may be the ultimate way of showing caring respect.

The question may be asked whether there are therapist variables which affect the outcome of family treatment which are specific to the practice of family therapy. Or, this question might be phrased, "In what ways is an effective family therapist different from an effective individual psychotherapist, psychoanalyst, group therapist, behavior therapist, and so on?" The meager research literature which speaks to the question of what constitutes an effective family therapist, for the most part, addresses the very same types of therapist variables that have been studied doggedly now for three decades in research on individual psychotherapy (cf: Gurman & Razin, 1977). Authors such as Tomm and Wright (1979), in their classic paper on the types of perceptual, conceptual and technical skill needed to be developed in the training of family therapists, suggest that there are, indeed, very specific skills which an effective family therapist must possess, some of which can be assessed outside of the therapeutic process, others of which can only be measured in the therapeutic process. Such therapist skills which are probably unique to practicing effective family therapy cannot afford to be assumed, but require empirical scrutiny.

LOOKING AHEAD:
CLOSING THE CLINICIAN-RESEARCHER GAP

So, what is an effective family therapist?—the words of Mark Twain reappear hauntingly and uncomfortably, "I was gratified to be able to answer promptly, and I did. I said I didn't know."

Perhaps the main reason why I do not know, and the field does not know, the answer to this question, is that we have been asking the wrong questions. This "wrong" question is the very one a handful of researchers have been trying to answer the last few years, and the evidence about which I have briefly reviewed thus far.

The medical historian Garrison wrote,

Whenever many different remedies are proposed for a disease, it usually means that we know very little about the disease, which is also true of a . . . (remedy) when it is vaunted as a panacea or cure-all for many diseases.

In keeping with Garrison's view, we may say that,

Whenever many different attributes and skills are proposed to characterize the effective family therapist, it usually means that we know very little about the effective family therapist, which is also true of a narrow range of therapist attributes and skills when they are vaunted as necessary and sufficient conditions for most methods of family therapy.

There probably exist a cluster of therapist characteristics of the "mensch" variety that can be shown to be functionally necessary, as minimal conditions, for the effective practice of all, or nearly all, methods of family therapy. What is equally likely, in my view, is that some of the characteristics of effective family therapists are quite different in different therapeutic approaches. In effect, rather different therapist "selves" may be required by different therapeutic methods. While continued investigation of therapist factors that make a difference across the "schools" of family therapy is certain to be of value, e.g., in the selection of family therapy trainees, it may be that extensive study of those therapist variables contribute heavily to outcomes *within* the different major "schools" of family therapy are likely to have greater ultimate practical relevance, and are likely to have more impact on the growth and continuing refinement of the practice of family therapy.

There has been a strong trend, at least in the United States, toward what has come to be known as the "clinical trial" approach to psychotherapy research. In this approach, therapist differences are held to a minimum, and the emphasis is on the differential effects on outcome of differing methods of psychotherapy *qua* methods. These so-called "comparative" studies are what Klein and Gurman (1981) have labelled, "comparative-competitive" studies. Ingenuine public statements of the rationale for such studies typically emphasize the aim of identifying which methods of therapy are best for which patients. Yet beneath the public patina of scientific objectivity and knowledge-seeking lurks an inevitable psychological truth: psychotherapy researchers, while they may not be normal, as Pittman (1981) noted, *are* human. Psychotherapy researchers always have a vested, and deeply personal, interest in the result of their studies. But such an understandable and very human desire to "find" that what is "best" is what one already believes in, has not been very helpful in convincing clinicians to change their ways on the basis of empirical evidence. Family therapists do not advocate different approaches based on their relative scientific status (Schwartz & Breunlin, 1983); they are attracted to different approaches on the basis of a large number of both rational and irrational factors (Gurman, 1983a). The choice of a favorite method of family therapy is sometimes healthy and sometimes pathological, but it is always very personal. For example, therapists with a "take charge" personal style may be better suited to Structural Family Therapy than to more reflective methods; therapists who prefer order and predictability may be more attracted to behavioral approaches; and Strategic therapists may be those who fear their own impotence, and so, require a team to let them do what they think is right. Psychodynamic therapists, of course, are those who were either born Jewish or believe that they should have been. As Skynner (1978) has quipped, we need "different thinks for different shrinks." The kind of research that most therapists will listen to is that which enhances the potency of the therapeutic approach to which the therapist is already deeply and personally committed. For those who will not commit themselves to anything, there is always the client-centered approach or, failing that, for physicians, the full time practice of psychopharmacology.

Thus, the way to ask the "right" questions on the matter of "what is an effective family therapist?" is to convert the conviction of each approach to family therapy into more precise questions, e.g., "What is the strength of the relationship between a therapist's level of differentiation and his outcome in Bowen therapy?"; "Are there reliable and strong correlations between the mental health of psychodynamically oriented family therapists and the outcomes they achieve, and on what sorts of criteria of mental health?"; "Can it be demonstrated that a therapist's predilection or capacity to think in non-linear terms affect the outcomes she achieves in practicing any of the variants of strategic family therapy (cf: Stanton, 1981)?"; "Does the therapist's openness to his/her own irrationality predict better outcomes in symbolic-experiential family therapy (Whitaker & Keith, 1981)?", and so on.

Data on these kinds of therapy-specific questions are the kinds to which workaday clinicians may actually listen. And, of those therapists who will not be influenced by data that contradict the tenets of the therapeutic religions to which they are loyal, it may be said that they suffer from chronic and severe Ideas of Reverence.

Research Designs, Circular Causality and the Effective Family Therapist

I would like to offer some thoughts about research designs for those family therapists who are not blocked by the Figments of their own Indoctrination. Just as systems theory and the so-called "new epistemology" have challenged virtually all the major assumptions of thinking in psychotherapy, the new breed of cybernetic family therapists have also begun to question the appropriateness of traditional research designs as well (cf: Gurman, 1983b; Tomm, 1983). As systems theory has taught us, a part can be understood in isolation from the whole (Keeney, 1983) only to a limited degree. This fundamental tenet requires us to ask whether it is possible to conceive meaningfully of the therapist's attributes and skills as "independent" variables. Paul Watzlawick once said that "Statistics are like bikinis: what they reveal is interesting, but what they conceal is vital." The same may be said of experimental designs in psychotherapy research, in which a particular variable, or set of variables, is varied in amount or degree. Thus, a class of therapists behaviors such as empathic responding, reframing the meaning of the identified patient's symptom, or blocking family members' usual maladaptive interaction, may be varied according to a research protocol, but in ways which, if adhered to strictly, could create ludicrous clinical situations: imagine a therapist being required to hold back empathy as a woman in marital therapy is painfully re-experiencing her rage at her father who physically abused her as a child.

The family therapist is necessarily a part of a circularly causal therapeutic system. But, "to the degree that the therapist is clear about the therapeutic task and is able to remain in 'role,' his/her behavior will be *responsive to*, but not controlled by, the (family) . . . While sensitive and reactive to the (family) and the environmental context, the therapist may function in what seems to be an independent and self determined manner" (Parloff et al., 1978). Ferreira (Framo, 1981) has noted, that "We had to recognize that the family was a system before we could recognize that the family does not always act like a system." We all know that while the family therapist is part of the therapeutic system, she must not become swallowed up by the family system, if she is to be effective.

At its extreme, the notion of circular causality has led, at times, to unfortunate denials that it is the responsibility of the family therapist to bring about change in families. Williamson (1981) has noted wryly,

> With linear causality, at least one knew at whom to point and about what to feel indignant. But now since the buck is in constant circulation it stops nowhere. Therefore, responsibility for behavior can be located nowhere. If responsibility for behavior is nowhere-then where can one look for change?" (p. 447)

While the complex processes of family therapy, viewed as a whole, are necessarily circular, subprocesses in the therapeutic encounter can be shown to be decidedly linear. Indeed, if this were not the case, then therapists should have no right to collect fees for their services: perhaps the therapist might collect a fee after each session, then immediately hand it back to the family. On alternating weeks, of course, the patient would first pay the family for their attendance, then, have his money returned to him (Gurman, 1983a).

Beavers (1979) has noted that "Communicating in a linear fashion allows us to be distinguished from the mad." While the sort of reductionism that has characterized much of psychotherapy research, including family therapy research, has often led to trivialization, it is important to bear in mind that "reductionism and wholism are complementary forms of description" (Keeney, 1983). The goal then, as Maslow (1970) has suggested becomes thinking "both about particulars and about wholes without falling into either meaningless particularism or vague and useless generality" (p. 317).

What, then, are the implications of this dialectical view for how to increase most appropriately our understanding of what an effective family therapist *is*, and what an effective family therapist *does*, that defines her as effective?

First, traditional models of research on the study of the family therapist's contribution to effective treatment are not precluded by adopting a systemic perspective on what occurs during therapy (Gurman, 1983a). Therapists offering given method of family therapy, within a research protocol, must first be rigorously trained in the method. Implementation checks on the therapist's behavior during therapy must establish with certainty that each therapist is conducting therapy in accordance with the principles of and guidelines for the conduct of that method, and must establish that each therapist is not doing things which the method defines as incompatible with, or unnecessary for, effective practice of the method. Moreover, each therapist must be shown to be competent in the method, before treating families in the formal study. Measures of stable therapist characteristics believed to influence the outcome of the therapy method can also be taken.

In such an approach, the search for circularly causal patterns that are associated with outcome comes not from the design of the study, but from data analysis. This approach is equally relevant to both controlled studies of the comparative efficacy of different therapies and to quasi-experimental designs applied to the study of only a single therapeutic method. In this approach, there is weight given to both the confirmatory aims of controlled research, and to the aim of discovery.

What is needed is not "outcome" studies or "process" studies; what is needed are process-outcome studies (Gurman, Kniskern & Pinsof, 1986). The study of therapeutic process alone, while valuable for examining certain theoretical propositions, is of limited utility unless it is paired with the assessment of clinical outcomes. Conversely, findings gathered in the more common scenario of studying the efficacy of a method of family therapy without examining in detail the processes involved in its application will usually fall on the deaf ears of clinicians (who are usually rather attentive types).

Naturalistic, correlational process-outcome analyses of the data gathered even in controlled comparative studies are called for. All of the variables involved in the technical operations of the therapist, as defined within a particular method of therapy, could be subjected to multivariate correlational analyses which would consider the relative contribution of each therapist variable to the overall pattern of outcome, or to specific target outcomes. It would also be possible to identify combinations, sequences, or patterns of therapist activity that are better predictors of outcome than any one therapist activity alone. Discriminant analyses, multiple regression analyses, or techniques such as path analysis, that consider temporal sequences, would be appropriate (Klein & Gurman, 1981).

Such a process-outcome investigative model is decidedly ecumenical and non-partisan. It assumes, in a way that is probably uncomfortable for many theorists of family therapy, that treatment theories do not always enumerate all of their operative principles, or active therapist ingredients, in their way of working. It also assumes that such principles and ingredients readily cross theoretical boundaries. It also assumes that some technical operations and therapist characteristics may be potent wherever they occur, even when they appear outside of their original theoretical framework for therapy. And, finally, it assumes that every method of family therapy contains prescriptions about who can practice the method effectively, and how to practice the method effectively which, in fact, are of little or no actual consequence to the efficacy of the method.

In brief, the identification of the effective family therapist requires that researchers simultaneously know very clearly what they are looking to find out, and be open to the possibility, indeed, likelihood, that they will find out things that they, or others, really did not want to know. Indeed, this is not an inaccurate way of characterizing the everyday work of family therapists as well.

REFERENCES

Alexander, J., & Parsons, B.V. (1973). Short-term behavioral intervention with delinquent families: Impact on family process and recidivism. *Journal of Abnormal Psychology, 81,* 219-255.

Alexander, J., Barton, C., Schiavo, R.S., & Parsons, B.V. (1976). Systems-behavioral intervention with families of delinquents: Therapist characteristics, family behavior and outcome. *Journal of Consulting and Clinical Psychology, 44,* 656-664.

Beavers, W.R. (1979). Personal communication.

Budman, S. & Shapiro, R. (1976). *Patients' evaluations of successful outcome in family and individual therapy.* Unpublished manuscript, University of Rochester Medical School

DeChenne, T.K. (1973). Experiential facilitation in conjoint marriage counseling. *Psychotherapy: Theory, Research and Practice, 10,* 212-214.

Framo, J.L. (1981). The integration of marital therapy with sessions with family of origin. In A. Gurman & D. Kniskern (Eds.), *Handbook of family therapy.* New York: Brunner/Mazel.

Freeman, S.J.J., Leavens, E.J., & McCullouch, D.J. (1969). Factors associated with success or failure in marital counseling. *Family Coordinator, 18*, 125-128.

Graham, J.A. (1968). The effect of the use of counselor positive responses to positive perceptions of mate in marriage counseling. *Dissertation Abstracts International, 28*, 2504A.

Griffin, R.W. (1967). Change in perception of marital relationship as related to marriage counseling. *Dissertation Abstracts International, 27*, 3956A.

Gurman, A.S. (1974). Attitude change in marital therapy. *Journal of Family Counseling, 2*, 50-54.

Gurman, A.S. (1975). Some therapeutic implications of marital therapy research. In A. Gurman (Ed.), *Couples in conflict*. New York: Jason Aronson.

Gurman, A.S. (1981). Integrative marital therapy: Toward the development of an interpersonal approach. In S. Budman (Ed.), *Forms of brief therapy*. New York: Guilford.

Gurman, A.S. (1983a). Family therapy research and the "new epistemology." *Journal of Marital and Family Therapy, 9*, 227-234.

Gurman, A.S. (1983b). *Psychotherapy research and the practice of psychotherapy*. Presidential Address, Society for Psychotherapy Research, Sheffield, England.

Gurman, A.S. & Kniskern, D.P. (1978a). Deterioration in marital and family therapy: Empirical, clinical and conceptual issues. *Family Process, 17*, 3-20.

Gurman, A.S. & Kniskern, D.P. (1978b). Research on marital and family therapy: Progress, perspective and prospect. In S. Garfield & A. Bergin (Eds.), *Handbook of psychotherapy and behavior change*. Second edition. New York: Wiley.

Gurman, A.S. & Kniskern, D.P. (1981). Family therapy outcome research: Knowns and unknowns. In A. Gurman & D. Kniskern (Eds.), *Handbook of family therapy*. New York: Brunner/Mazel.

Gurman, A.S., Kniskern, D.P. & Pinsof, W.M. (1986). Research on the process and outcome of marital and family therapy. In S. Garfield & A. Bergin (Eds.), *Handbook of psychotherapy and behavior change*. Third edition. New York: Wiley.

Gurman, A.S. & Razin, A.M. (1977). *Effective psychotherapy: A handbook of research*. New York: Pergamon.

Haley, J. (1976). *Problem solving therapy*. San Francisco: Jossey-Bass.

Jones, B.S. (1969). Functions of meaning clarification by therapists in a psychotherapy group. *Dissertation Abstracts International, 29*, 3706A.

Keeney, B.P. (1983). *Aesthetics of change*. New York: Guilford.

Kerr, M. (1981). Family systems theory and therapy. In A. Gurman & D. Kniskern (Eds.), *Handbook of family therapy*. New York: Brunner/Mazel.

Klein, M.H. & Gurman, A.S. (1981). Ritual and reality: Some clinical implications of experimental design. In L.P. Rehm (Ed.), *Behavior therapy for depression*. New York: Academic Press.

Lorion, R. P. (1973). Socioeconomic status and traditional treatment approaches reconsidered. *Psychological Bulletin, 79*, 263-270.

Maslow, A. (1970). *Motivation and personality*. New York: Harper and Row.

McGoldrick, M., Pearce, J. & Giordano, J. (Eds.) (1982). *Ethnicity and family therapy*. New York: Guilford.

Parloff, M.B., Waskow, I.E. & Wolfe, B. (1978). Research on therapist variables in relation to process and outcome. In S. Garfield & A. Bergin (Eds.), *Handbook of psychotherapy and behavior change*. Second edition. New York: Wiley.

Pittman, F.S. (1981). The awards: An effort at justification. *American Family Therapy Association Newsletter*, Number 6 (October), 3-5.

Rabkin, J.G. (1977). Therapist's attitudes toward mental illness and health. In A. Gurman & A. Razin (Eds.), *Effective psychotherapy: A handbook of research*. New York: Pergamon.

Roberts, P.V. (1975). The effects on marital satisfaction of brief training in behavioral exchange negotiation medicated by differentially experienced trainers. *Dissertation Abstracts International, 36*, 457B.

Rice, D.G., Fey, W.F., & Kepecs, J.G. (1972). Therapist experience and "style" in co-therapy. *Family Process, 11*, 1-12.

Sager, C.J. (1981). Couples therapy and marriage contracts. In A. Gurman & D. Kniskern (Eds.), *Handbook of family therapy*. New York: Brunner/Mazel.

Santa-Barbara, K., Woodward, C., Levin, D., Goodman, J. & Epstein, N. (1975). *The relationship between therapists' characteristics and outcome variables in family therapy*. Paper presented at the Canadian Psychiatric Association Meeting, Banff, Alberta.

Sattler, J.M. (1977). The effects of therapist-client racial similarity. In A. Gurman & A. Razin (Eds.), *Effective psychotherapy: A handbook of research*. New York: Pergamon.

Schwartz, R.C. & Breunlin, D. (1983). Research: Why clinicians should bother with it. Family Therapy Newsletter, 7, 23-27, 57-59.

Shapiro, R. (1974) Therapist attitudes and premature termination in family and individual therapy. *Journal of Nervous and Mental Disease, 159,* 101-107.

Shapiro, R. & Budman, S. (1973). Defection, termination, and continuation in family and individual therapy. *Family Process, 12,* 55-67.

Shellow, R., Brown, B., & Osberg, J. (1963). Family group therapy in retrospect: Four years and sixty families. *Family Process, 2,* 52-67.

Schreiber, L. (1966). Evaluation of family group treatment in a family agency. *Family Process, 5,* 21-29.

Skynner, A.C.R. (1981). An open-systems, group analytic approach to family therapy. In A. Gurman, & D. Kniskern (Eds.), *Handbook of family therapy.* New York: Brunner/Mazel.

Skynner, A.C.R. (1978). Personal communication.

Stanton, M.D. (1981). Strategic approaches to family therapy. In A. Gurman & D. Kniskern (Eds.), *Handbook of family therapy.* New York: Brunner/Mazel.

Tomm, K. (1983). The old hat doesn't fit. *Family Therapy Networker, 7,* 39-41.

Tomm, K., & Wright, L. (1979). Training in family therapy: Perceptual, conceptual and executive skills. *Family Process, 18,* B27-250.

Waxenberg, B.R. (1973). Therapists' empathy, regard and genuineness as factors in staying in or dropping out of short-term, time-limited family therapy. *Dissertation Abstracts International, 34,* 1288B.

Woodward, C., Santa-Barbara, J., Levin, S., Goodman, J., Streiner, D. & Epstein, N. (1975). *Client and therapist characteristics related to family therapy outcome: Closure and follow-up evaluation.* Paper presented at the Society for Psychotherapy Research Meeting, Boston.

Whitaker, C.A., & Keith, D.V. (1981). Symbolic-experiential family therapy. In A. Gurman & D. Kniskern (Eds.), *Handbook of Family Therapy.* New York: Brunner/Mazel.

Williamson, D.S. (1981). Termination of the intergenerational boundary between first and second generations: A "new" stage in the family life cycle. *Journal of Marital and Family Therapy, 7,* 441-452.

Are All Therapists Alike?
Use of Self in Family Therapy:
A Multidimensional Perspective

Meri L. Shadley

ABSTRACT. Since most of the existing research within family therapy has been school-specific, a multidimensional viewpoint regarding use of self has been lacking. This study investigated how therapists from various theoretical orientations perceive and make use of themselves within therapeutic relationships. All the subjects confirmed that self-awareness is critical to clinical effectiveness and that the professional self cannot be separated from the personal self. As well, the qualities of genuineness, connection-making, encouragement, humor, respect, and trust were consistently relayed as important to clinical relationships. Finally, a continuum of self-disclosure styles was developed to portray the assorted dimensions related to use of self practices. Variations in these therapists' styles were primarily related to gender, and secondarily to theoretical orientation and clinical experience. Significant personal life events were frequently indicated as creating the largest amount of change in one's tendencies to use self intimately.

In a recent "dictionary" of family therapy terms and concepts, use of self was defined as "the therapist's feeling response to the family members" (Sauber, L'Abate, & Weeks, 1985, p. 173). The felt self is certainly one dimension of the therapist's processes, but additional responses include verbal or non-verbal expression of these feelings and personal self-disclosure.

A concise, but comprehensive, definition of the term "use of self" is presently missing from the field. Part of the reason for this inadequacy is that the therapist's use of self is a multifaceted and individualized phenomenon. For many, it is a process of accepting one's self as a fellow

Meri L. Shadley, M.A., is in private practice, 1022 Forest Street, Reno, NV 89509, and a doctoral student at Saybrook Institute in San Francisco, CA. Additionally, she has trained community professionals throughout the western states and is president-elect of the Nevada Association of Marriage and Family Therapy.

Acknowledgement is given to dissertation committee chairman, Dennis Jaffee, Ph.D., and member, Stanley Krippner, Ph.D., as well as colleague, Charles T. Holt, M.A., for feedback on this paper. Special thanks to Pru Jones for her invaluable assistance and encouragement throughout the data analysis of this study.

human who offers more than professional expertise. For others, acknowledging personal vulnerabilities and capabilities provides clarity about which parts of self to withhold in order to retain strength, health, and integrity. To understand and congruently use one's self, then, a therapist must consider various factors. Some of these influential factors are one's personality, personal and professional experiences and realities, theoretical orientation, and, of course, each interpersonal context.

Questions about the effect of these factors and appropriate use of self have long been discussed by individual and group therapists (Buber, 1970; Fagan, 1970; Kopp, 1972; Yalom, 1975). In family therapy, however, even though individuals such as Satir and Whitaker have consistently used their personhood in therapy, the field has only recently begun to explore the issue more directly (Aponte, 1982; Kramer, 1985).

Unfortunately, the existing adherence to school-specific approaches in family therapy research clouds our knowledge about commonalities and differences in our thinking and our practice. Integrative research, such as this study, may unveil important information about how the therapist's use of self is viewed and approached across the various family therapy orientations. As well, it may help clarify some of the important aspects critical to therapists learning to use themselves effectively.

METHODOLOGY

This multidimensional invetigation into family therapists' use of self was part of broad-based research on the professional development process. Semi-structured interviews of thirty (30) therapists from three regions of the United States were conducted during the fall of 1985. The subjects were solicited by obtaining referrals from a variety of family therapy training institutes and individual trainers. Because of the study's overall research goals, all interviewees had to have participated in some sort of formalized family therapy training.

The study was organized into three major sections—training experiences, personal/professional interface processes, and theories about clinical practice—with the interviews typically progressing chronologically. First, completion of a single page data sheet, and a brief personal genogram led to a discussion of how pretraining influences affected one's choice of family therapy orientation and particular training program. Second, subjects were asked questions about the type and usefulness of specific training activities. Third, parallel processes were explored in an attempt to understand how therapists transform learnings from their training experiences, clinical practice, and personal life situations into an evolving therapeutic style. Finally, the subject was asked to respond, on a scale of 1 to 10, to three randomly ordered questions.

Data Analysis Procedures

The researcher initially examined information from the taped interviews in an individual case format. Next, a matrix was developed to discover critical themes in experiences, opinions, perceptions, and practices. Due to the comprehensiveness of this study, only the responses specifically related to the use of self topic are detailed in this report.

Ratings on one of the scaled questions were reviewed along with responses to questions such as "How do you use yourself within therapeutic interactions?" Themes emerging from this and related data included: (1) therapist's definition and awareness of self, (2) qualities ascribed as critical to therapeutic relationships, (3) use of self dimensions and styles, and (4) critical events that lead to changes in use of self styles.

Demographics

An attempt was made to solicit a cross-section of therapists, but the interviewed subjects are not meant to be a representative sample of the entire family therapy field. Of the 17 female and 13 male therapists interviewed, 10 lived on the west coast (San Francisco or Reno, Nevada), 11 on the east coast (New York and Boston vicinities), and 9 in the greater Chicago area.

The age range was from 31 to 65, with a mean age of 41 and a median age of 38. Sixty percent were in their first marriage and had two or more children, while 8 had no children and 3 had never been married.

Although the interviewed therapists came from 19 diverse training experiences, no more than 4 individuals came from any one program. Six subjects had been out of their specialized family therapy training for three to four years, 13 for five to six years, 6 for seven to nine years ago, and 5 for ten to fifteen years.

RESULTS

While many family therapy orientations originated from one of the basic philosophical stances within psychology, the incorporation of systems concepts has created new terms to explain the way family therapists describe their work. It is interesting to note, however, that most of the therapists interviewed in this study stated that the process of defining their therapeutic orientation was quite difficult. Only those using the terms "Bowen systems," "structural/strategic," and "eclectic" did not hesitate in their terminology. Other words used in various combinations were integrative, communications, systemic, psychodynamic, and psychoanalytic.

Despite the different combinations clearly indicating diversity in the family therapy field, meaningful classification is impossible to ascertain. Because the numbers are too small if a more specialized categorizational system is used, the researcher organized the orientations into general groupings. The demographic factors of age, geographical location, degree, and marital status were compatible within the categories. The four groupings are as follows:

— *Purist*: The 8 interviewees (6 female, 2 male) who indicated only one specific family therapy school or well-known leader's orientation. (e.g., structural, Satir communications, Bowen systems, integrative, etc.).
— *Structural/Strategic Blend*: The 8 subjects (2 female, 6 male) who labeled their orientation as a blend of the structural and strategic family therapy schools.
— *Integrational Blend*: The 7 interviewees (5 female, 2 male) who used a label or description indicating a combination of any two therapeutic philosophies other than structural/strategic. (e.g., integrative/structural, structural/communications, strategic/Bowen, etc.).
— *Eclectic*: The 7 therapists (4 female, 3 male) who either used this specific term or who named a minimum of three separate family schools to describe their orientation. (e.g., Bowen and structural/strategic, or psychodynamic/integrative/strategic).

Therapist's Definition and Awareness of Self

To better understand how family therapists view the use of self, the researcher initially inquired, "What is the self of the family therapist?" Within each personalized definition, interviewees typically included a variation of one of the following phrases: "all systems interacting," "everything within a dynamic interplay," "all life's experiences transformed," "patterns formed by past, present, and future," "natural responsiveness to each context," "integration of total person," "integrity of all self parts," and "the essence of who or what I am as a person." Even with the slight variations noted above, this researcher's definition of the professional self as a "constantly evolving system that is changed by the conscious and unconscious interplay of the numerous systems impacting the clinician" appears confirmed by the subjects definitions. The interviewees were not asked directly, yet all but one indicated their professional and personal selves to be intricately intertwined and not separable into distinct entities.

Subjects' responses to the scaled statement "I believe that awareness of my self is a very important ingredient in my effectiveness as a family therapist'' indicate an extremely high agreement (9.6 average on a scale of 1 to 10) with the idea of therapists' remaining mindful of self. More than 75% of the subjects rated the statement a ten, and all ratings were at least an eight. Even though it might be interesting (and more dramatic) to focus on the slight variations found, these results primarily confirm the existence of a commonality within the field.

Critical Aspects of Therapeutic Relationships

Based upon Carl Whitaker's belief that the self ''gains in definition and potential'' when it is in ''communion with others in relationship'' (Neill & Kniskern, 1982, p. 20), another relevant question is: ''What personal qualities are critical to one's use of self within therapeutic relationships?'' This question referred to qualities of the therapist's own style of being with clients, but many of the subjects included qualities that came out of the therapeutic situation itself. Thus, the interface of therapist's qualities and qualities of the therapeutic situation are interwoven within these results.

The information given by the subjects falls into nine categories. The first four—empathy, warmth, humor, and genuineness—are well known qualities that have been found to be highly related to positive clinical outcomes (Alexander, Barton, Schiavo, & Parsons, 1976; Gurman & Kniskern, 1978). The additional aspects—respect, trust, connection, encouragement, and objectivity—were determined by reviewing other interviewee comments. Their observations were then organized into the five categories as follows:

— *Connection*: attachment, resonate, be part of a whole with the family, invest oneself, open one's self to pain;
— *Encouragement:* challenge, confront, enable, wants success, push for goals, desire movement;
— *Trust:* create safe environment, go with the flow, using one's intuitiveness, sensing the spiritual relationship
— *Respect:* being awed or inspired by the client family's resilience, politeness, not provoke intensity unnecessarily;
— *Objectivity:* setting limits, maintaining distance, reserved, being selective, wanting another's picture or view.

The interview dialogues frequently indicated the same category several times, yet most of the therapists found two or three categories particularly valuable to their use of self. Overall, when the nine categories were analyzed from most to least referenced, five clusters were found: (1) genuineness and connection, (2) encouragement and humor, (3) trust and respect, (4) empathy and warmth, and (5) objectivity. The third and fourth clusters, while equal in number of references, were found to be of varying importance to the different orientations. Some of the more specific results are detailed below.

First, therapists from all orientations found genuineness to be one of the most important qualities to effective use of self. Both the purist and the eclectic groupings, in fact, were nearly twice as likely to indicate genuineness and connection above all other qualities. The structural/strategic blend therapists, however, talked of trust and encouragement and the integrational blend group mentioned humor and respect most often.

Second, a particularly important difference was found between genders within the structural/strategic blend orientation. The cluster of respect and trust was highly significant to the male therapists, but a combination of humor, encouragement, and genuineness was of primary importance to the females.

Also of interest was the finding that women therapists within the purist grouping referenced the quality of connection more often than either their male counterparts or women from the other theoretical orientations.

Finally, very few of the subjects ended up mentioning any of the objectivity categorized statements without making an additional comment. One of the subjects, for example, stated that she typically was "reserved, but connected."

Dimensions of Self-Disclosure

If the therapist's use of self is as much a technique as it is a quality of relating, then it is important to begin looking at how various therapists actually make use of this "prime instrument" (Kramer, 1985). What and how thoughts, feelings, and actions are incorporated into one's therapeutic style are critical to understanding and facilitating this development. The question, "How do you use yourself within your therapeutic interactions?" elicited many responses around the theme of sharing one's self with client families. Specific dimensions within self-disclosure emerged as the researcher searched for patterns in use of self styles.

One dimension continually referenced was verbal versus non-verbal disclosures of who the therapist was as a "real" person. Most of the subjects felt that paralleling their own life with the client family's life was a useful strategy, but several stated they did not always feel comfortable with verbal references. For example, one therapist felt that since she and her husband worked out of their home, a great deal of her personal life was already revealed. It was her premise that important parallel's could already be seen through the environmental situation and more specific information might best be left unsaid.

Conversely, some non-visible parallels were more typically shared with clients than others. Examples of commonly shared parallels were the therapist's struggles with being the oldest sibling, being a stepparent, caring for an ill parent or a new baby, dealing with conflicting responsibilities, and personal or professional transitions. Few subjects mentioned interactional examples. Apparently, therapists are more likely to openly discuss individual parallels than relationship parallels.

Those who did talk of personal relationship examples began to delineate another important dimension. These subjects frequently discussed their comfort with relaying present versus past personal issues. Some felt that sharing current situations was "too hard, emotionally," while others felt that such sharing helped them to be less encumbered by their corresponding personal or professional issues. Most subjects, however, agreed that sharing relevant past information was usually very effective without being too personally distressful.

If interviewees did not tend to share either past or present personal facts with their clients, they typically talked of several other ways of using their selves within therapeutic relationships. Some spoke of sharing their impressions, opinions and/or feelings regarding the client's situation, whereas others stated that they frequently used movies, television programs, books, friend's or other client's situations, and anecdotes to parallel and/or relate to client families. Other interviewees share their personal reactions to the therapeutic relationship itself. Some of these therapists discussed their freedom to share "here and now" emotions such as tears and laughter. Again, many felt comfortable sharing themselves overtly, and others believed that they were able to convey these reactions through "unspoken emotional arms."

Use of Self Styles

Based upon the dimensions detailed above, a continuum of self-disclosure styles was delineated.

— *Intimate interaction*: Tends to share self through verbal and non-verbal expressions of therapeutic reactions. References to present or past personal issues are likely.
— *Reactive response*: Typically expresses both non-verbal and verbal feelings of emotional connectedness within therapeutic relationships, but generally does not verbalize personal life details or parallels.
— *Controlled response*: Inclined to maintain a slight distance by limiting self-disclosures to past experiences, non-verbalized feelings, anecdotes, or literary parallels.
— *Reflective feedback*: The exposure of self through questioning or challenging families and by giving impressions. Seldom shares personal information or strong emotional reactions.

These four descriptions indicate distinctions among styles, therefore, it may be helpful to view them as forming a continuum from most to least personally self-disclosive. Use of such a continuum implies that, depending on the context, therapists actually use a combination or variety of styles. From their discussions, however, a predominant style was indicated and thus attributed to each interviewee.

When looking at self-disclosure styles across the demographic factors of training program attended, degree, marital status, and parenting status, it appeared that all styles were represented. Specific differences were found when viewing these styles across therapeutic orientation, gender, and clinical experience.

Male therapists within the structural/strategic blend orientation were the only group to indicate a high usage of the reflective feedback style. Therapists within the purists and the integrational blend groupings appeared to favor the controlled response and the reactive response styles. True to the name eclectic, therapists from this grouping indicated an equal distribution of self-disclosure styles.

The most interesting difference was that while the majority of males (62%) were found to use the controlled response or reflective feedback style of self-disclosure, more females (65%) used the reactive response or intimate interaction styles. Only one man indicated that he responded primarily within the intimate interaction style and only one woman within the reflective feedback style. The woman stated that her style appeared to be changing towards more direct intimacy.

Finally, several differences were found when these self-disclosure styles were related to the therapists' clinical experience. (1) All therapists with less than seven years experience indicated either a controlled response or reflective feedback style. (2) Male therapists categorized in the controlled response style averaged 10 years experience, but those in the other styles averaged 8 years. (3) Female therapists indicating either an intimate interaction or reflective response style averaged 11 years experience, while those indicating a controlled response or reflective feedback style averaged six years. These results suggest that there may be a personal/professional development aspect related to self-disclosure styles.

Critical Events Effecting Use of Self Styles

A major focus of the interview was to determine interface issues within therapists' professional and personal lives, yet it was still surprising to discover that personal transitions and/or tragedies were the most likely circumstances to induce therapeutic style changes. Numerous factors affected how these family therapists made clinical use of themselves as persons, but some specific life and death events within their own immediate family were typically mentioned as having the strongest impact.

Having children, for example, pushed some therapists to withhold more of their energy in therapy so they could handle the pressures of both personal and professional relationships. Several subjects mentioned that this distancing allowed them to be more understanding and patient of others as well as less critical and competitive with themselves. As well, many subjects stated that being a parent gave them more freedom to self-disclose and to feel more comfortable with their own idiosyncracies.

The death of a parent (or parent figure) was also described as particularly significant to changes in therapeutic style. As might be expected, therapists experiencing these personal losses became much more interested in building a client family's relationships than solving their problems. Several interviewees stated that their way of being with clients also became much more emotionally intimate than it had been previously.

Interviewed therapists mentioned that other factors impacted the way in which they used themselves as people, but no other factors were discussed as frequently or by as broad a range of the subjects. Additional factors included training and clinical experiences, being in therapy oneself, personal transitions such as divorce, disengagement from family of origin, children leaving home, and one's developmental life cycle.

SUMMARY AND DISCUSSION

In searching for similarities and differences in various family therapist's use of self, this investigation discovered more commonalities within the field than has been indicated by previous school-specific research. For example, along with the well-known relationship aspects of empathy, warmth, humor, and genuineness; connection, encouragement, and respect were invariably mentioned as critical to forming trusting interactions with client families. Therapists, no matter what their orientation, believed that an assortment of these therapeutic qualities were conducive to effective use of self. As well, a variety of therapists discussed similar issues when describing dimensions important to their comfortable use of self-disclosure. Other consistently held beliefs were that the personal and professional selves are interwoven and that self-awareness is very important to being a competent family therapist.

From this study's small sample of a cross-section of clinicians, theoretical orientation appears to be only one of several critical factors contributing to a therapist's use of self. Gender, the amount of clinical experience, and significant life events also play an important role in therapeutic style.

The most outstanding result of this study is that gender, rather than theoretical orientation, has the strongest impact upon the way in which therapists' make use of themselves in their therapeutic relationships. No matter what label they used to describe their orientation, female interviewees were more likely to use personal life examples and/or present feelings with client families. Males, on the other hand, frequently focused on other people's feelings and situations when relating to or paralleling their clients' experiences.

These gender differences were particularly significant when structural/strategic blend oriented therapists were compared. Not only do female therapists within this orientation value the quality of genuineness more highly than their male counterparts, but they are much more likely to use an openly revealing self-disclosure style. Although the number of females within this theoretical orientation was much smaller than the number of males, the regularity of these variations imply definite stylistic differences. These results, along with the general outcomes mentioned above, confirm recent contentions within the family therapy field regarding important male/female differences.

The results related to amount of clinical experience and use of self are preliminary findings due to the lack of therapists with more varied experience levels. The findings, however, tentatively indicate a possible developmental aspect related to styles of therapeutic self-disclosure. One advanced therapist's statement, "I use me more now, but in some ways that is less" suggests an interesting way of looking at use of self that demands more exploration.

While some professional experiences were discussed, the personal life events of becoming a parent or losing a significant loved one was more frequently mentioned as having a strong influence on changes in one's professional direction and therapeutic style. It appeared from the interviews that these major transitions and/or tragedies were likely to compel therapists into closer and more intimate contact with their client families.

To accurately interpret the findings from this introductory study, methodological problems must be taken into account. Some of the major difficulties are:

1. the small, non-representative sample of family therapists (MD's, "master" therapists, and pure strategically-oriented therapists are missing from the sample.);
2. the non-specific organization of the various orientations; and
3. the imbalance of male and female subjects within the four orientation groupings.

Based upon the interesting results that did emerge from this initial study, further research with a larger number of varying and more specifically-oriented therapists is certainly warranted. Such a study would allow for a more detailed exploration into the factors incorporated in and affecting therapist's use of self.

In the meantime, however, these results suggest that family therapy training programs may want to include methods for assisting trainees to become aware of and integrate their emerging professional self into a flexible, personalized use of self style.

REFERENCES

Alexander, J., Barton, C., Schiavo, R., & Parsons, B. (1976). Systems-behavioral intervention with families of delinquents: Therapist characteristics, family behavior and outcome. *Journal of Consulting and Clinical Psychology, 44,* 656-664.

Aponte, H. J. (1982). The person of the therapist: The cornerstone of therapy. *The Family Therapy Networker, 6* (2), 19-21, 46.

Buber, M. (1970). *I and thou.* New York: Charles Scribner's Sons.

Fagan, J. (1970). The tasks of the therapist. In J. Fagan & I. L. Shepherd (Eds.), *Gestalt therapy now: Theory, techniques, applications* (pp. 88-106). Palo Alto, CA: Science and Behavior Books.

Gurman, A. S., & Kniskern, D. P. (1978). Research on marital and family therapy: Progress, perspective and prospect. In S. Garfield & A. Bergin (Eds.), *Handbook of psychotherapy and behavior change.* New York: Wiley.

Kopp, S. B. (1972). *If you meet the Buddha on the road, kill him.* Palo Alto, CA: Science and Behavior Books.

Kramer, J. (1985). *Family interfaces: Transgenerational patterns.* New York: Brunner/Mazel.

Neill, J. R., & Kniskern, D. P. (Eds.). (1982). *From psyche to system: The evolving therapy of Carl Whitaker.* New York: Guilford Press.

Sauber, S. R., L'Abate, L., & Weeks, G. R. (1985). *Family therapy: Basic concepts and terms.* Rockville, MD: Aspen Publications.

Yalom, I. D. (1975). *The theory and practice of group psychotherapy.* New York: Basic Books.

Implications of the Wounded-Healer Paradigm for the Use of the Self in Therapy

Grant D. Miller
DeWitt C. Baldwin Jr.

ABSTRACT. The use of the self in therapy relates closely to the paradigm of the wounded-healer. The paradigm holds that deep within each healer lies an inner wound which may not only play an important role in vocational choice, but constitute a significant if not essential factor contributing to healing in the patient. Its mythical origins are described along with a diagrammatic model which attempts to analyze the interactional dynamics in the healer-patient encounter.

INTRODUCTION

It is clear that the therapeutic situation has the capacity to activate greater power and complexity than can be accounted for by the mere physical presence of the therapist in individual, family, and group therapy. Some of this mysterious power clearly is a function of role and charisma. From time immemorial, the healer[1] has achieved his place in society by means of special knowledge, training and skills not ordinarily available to other members of society. Additional personal qualities probably function to motivate certain persons to become healers and to generate the charismatic power frequently attributed to this role and to such persons. At the same time, an important contribution to the equation comes from the patient,[1] whose pain, suffering and need create a readiness to ascribe such power to another person in the hope and expectation of help. The nature of these hopes and expectations, as well as the corresponding role of the healer in a particular society or period of history has varied widely along an activity-passivity continuum (Fink, 1979).

Grant D. Miller, M.D., is Assistant Dean for Student Affairs and Associate Professor, Department of Psychiatry and Behavioral Sciences at the University of Nevada School of Medicine, Reno, NV 89557-0046.

DeWitt C. Baldwin Jr., M.D., is Director of the Office of Education Research of the American Medical Association, 535 North Dearborn Street, Chicago, IL 60610, and Adjunct Professor of Health Professions Education at the Center for Educational Development, University of Illinois, Chicago, IL.

It is not in the purpose of this article to prescribe the role and behavior of the healer. However, we clearly assume and favor a positive, trusting relationship in which the healer genuinely interacts with a person in need, conveys warmth and empathy in a nonpossessive fashion, and attempts to grasp the meaning of the other person's life and experience in an effort to create an environment of safety and acceptance (Yalom, 1980). It is our view that the healer must not only create such an environment, but must be and act in such a way as to release and enhance the inherent healing powers of the patient.

How does this view relate to the use of the self in therapy? We propose that the nature of the helping relationship embodies the basic polarities inherent in the paradigm of the wounded-healer.[2] These polarities ultimately relate to the vulnerability and healing power in both healer and patient. The wounded-healer paradigm presented here emphasizes the potential of the healer's vulnerable or wounded side to release such power in the therapeutic relationship. This paper, then, will examine the paradigm of the wounded-healer in historical perspective, present a conceptual and diagrammatic model of the helping relationship, and finally, spell out the implications of this paradigm for the use of the self in therapy.

POLARITIES

Fascination with the polarities of life is as old as recorded time. In his earliest statements, man refers to the contradictions of life and death, light and dark, and health and illness. In fact, the myths of many cultures refer to dieties in terms of such properties. The Babylonian dog goddess was called Gula as death and Labartu as healing. In India, Kali was both the goddess of the pox as well as the healer.

In Plato's Symposium (Hamilton, 1951), Aristophanes recounts an ancient myth which represented the earliest human beings as possessing four arms and legs, with one head and two faces, each looking in opposite directions. These beings supposedly possessed such qualities and intelligence that they caused fear and envy in the gods, resulting in the spheres being cut in half in order to reduce their power. Since then, the severed parts have endeavored to reunite in order to know, even for a moment, the ecstasy of reunification and wholeness. Indeed, the attempt to balance polarities lies at the heart of most of man's efforts to understand his place in the cosmos (Meyerhoff, 1976).

THE MYTH OF THE WOUNDED-HEALER

In the context of polarity, the concept of the wounded-healer takes on a powerful meaning for the helping professions. Indeed, the paradox of one who heals and yet remains wounded lies at the heart of the mystery of healing. As with polarities, there is a long history to the concept of the wounded-healer which is stated clearly in the myth of Asclepius and Chiron (Graves, 1955). Asclepius is born of the union of the god Apollo and the mortal woman Coronis. During her pregnancy, Coronis is killed by Apollo's sister, Artemis, when it is discovered that Coronis has been unfaithful to Apollo. While Coronis is on the funeral pyre, Apollo snatches Asclepius from her womb, and gives him to the centaur healer, Chiron, to raise. Paradoxically, Chiron suffers from an incurable wound originally caused by the poisoned arrows of Hercules. Thus, Chiron is a healer who needs healing himself. Kerenyi (1959, pp. 96-97) comments: "all in all, Chiron, the wounded divine physician . . . seems to be the most contradictory figure in all Greek mythology. Although he is a Greek god, he suffers an incurable wound. Moreover, his nature combines the animal and Apollonian, for despite his horse's body, mark of the fecund and destructive creatures of nature that centaurs are otherwise known to be, he instructs heroes in medicine and music." Under Chiron's tutelage, Asclepius becomes the Greek god of healing.

The image of the wounded-healer is found again in the medieval myth of Parsifal. In the account of Chretien de Troye, the Fisher King, despite possessing the Holy Grail which grants all things to all persons, suffers interminably from an incurable wound (Johnson, 1977). The Fisher King is unable to avail himself of its cure for his own wound, but instead must wait until the liberation of the Holy Grail by Parsifal.

Equally rooted in our past is the tradition of the shaman, the primitive healer who, in most societies, is not only medicine man but priest (Harner, 1980; Meyerhoff, 1976). The shaman is able to have direct contact with the gods and spirits; experiences heaven, hell and the world, and stands at the junction of the opposing forces of life and death. He enters into and takes on the wounds and illnesses of his people, trancending these by his force and power. In many ways, the shaman is a wounded-healer in the fullest sense.

RECENT INTEREST
IN THE WOUNDED-HEALER PARADIGM

More recently, interest in the paradigm of the wounded-healer has experienced a revival among Jung and his followers, perhaps because of their interest in polarities, mythology and archetypes. Jung (1951) refers to the wounded-healer paradox when he states, "Only the wounded doctor can heal," while Guggenbuhl-Craig (1971) maintains that a healer-patient archetype exists and is activated each time a person becomes ill. In his view, each patient has an inner healer. However, when the intra-psychic or inner healer does not act to heal the patient, the sick person may seek an external healer. Not only does the patient have a hidden inner healer, but the healer has a hidden inner patient, and healer and patient frequently cast mutual projections upon each other based on their hidden parts. As elaborated by Groesbeck (1975, pp. 127-128), the process goes as follows: "The patient who is ill looks for an outer healer [who] looks for patients, as that is his vocation . . . . Because of his illness, the patient activates his 'inner . . . healer.'" This inner healer, however, is not integrated into consciousness, but is projected onto and constellated in the outer person of the healer. So too, the healer's own vulnerability, as reflected in unresolved emotional or somatic illnesses, is activated by his contact with the sick person. This largely unconscious, opposite pole of the archetypal image is projected onto the patient, rather than being integrated. Groesbeck continues: "if the relationship remains like this, no movement to a real cure occurs though outward remedies, physical and psychological, are applied. Real cure can only take place if the patient gets in touch with and receives help from his 'inner healer.' And this can only happen if the projections . . . are withdrawn." Hence, the healer must be in touch with and be aware of his own wounded side, if these projections are to be withdrawn. If the projections remain, both healer and patient attempt to manipulate the other to conform to inner need.

A MODEL FOR VIEWING THE HEALING PROCESS

Groesbeck (1975) includes several useful diagrams in his paper describing the archetypal image of the wounded-healer. Figure 1 represents a composite of these with numbered arrows representing both positive and negative interactions affecting the healing relationship. Examples are included to provide clarification.

In Arrow 1, the patient becomes wounded by one or more problems faced in human existence. The discomfort and pain experienced by the wounded patient stimulates a conscious search for help. A large number of factors are typically considered in choosing a particular healer, but many of these contribute little to healing. For example, an individual or family may seek therapy from a well-known and charismatic psychotherapist, but unless certain ingredients to be listed below are present in the therapeutic relationship, healing may not occur.

The healer with his professional training, licenses, experience, and popularity, consciously and objectively deals with the wounds of the patient (Arrow 2). The presence of the wound in the patient causes an emotional and/or physical imbalance which activates the wounded-healer polarity (Arrow 3) and a strong wish to be healed and return to health. Like metal shavings drawn to a magnet, attention to the discomfort of the wound bars the patient from conscious awareness of the healer within himself (Arrow 4). The inner healer polarity of the patient, then, is disregarded and is projected onto or identified within the outer professional healer (Arrow 5).

WOUNDED-HEALER PARADIGM

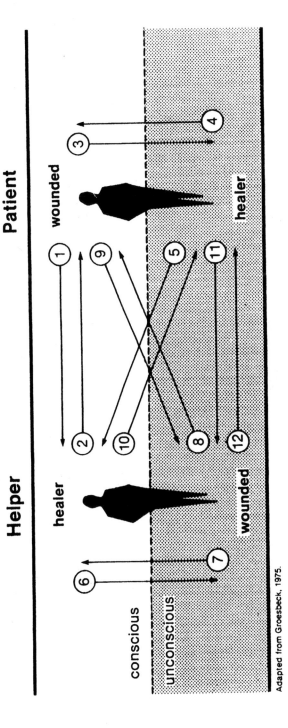

FIGURE 1. Diagram of the Wounded-Healer Paradigm

Adapted from Groesbeck, 1975.

143

Although all patients project their inner healer onto the professional healer to a certain degree, certain individuals do this to an extreme. Dependent individuals emphasize the importance of the professional healer through passively relinquishing their responsibility. Occasionally, flattery is used to maintain such a relationship, which not only inhibits healing, but tends to reinforce the projections of the professional healer.

The approach of a wounded individual for treatment also activates the wounded-healer polarity within the helper (Arrow 6). If the wounded pole is not experienced or integrated by the healer (Arrow 7), the wound is likely to be solely identified in or projected onto the patient (Arrow 8). Projection of healer wounds onto the patient (Arrow 8) is largely unconscious and is likely to occur in a number of circumstances, especially if both helper and patient have something in common and consciously or unconsciously identify with each other. In such a case, treatment may be compromised through loss of professional objectivity.

The following case example illustrates problems which may occur (Arrow 8). During the first year of an internal medicine residency, a resident whose father was an alcoholic, was observed to deal harshly with patients having alcohol-related physical problems. He was overheard saying: "You chose to drink which eventually led to this problem; so don't expect me to prescribe much pain medication." In this case, anger toward the resident's alcoholic father was inappropriately displaced and projected onto the alcoholic patient.

Both of the authors have suffered chronic illnesses and are literally wounded, perhaps partially explaining our mutual interest in the wounded-healer paradigm. One author has had diabetes for over 25 years. As a diabetic physician approached for care by a diabetic patient, this author must be aware of a bewildering number of feelings (Arrow 8). Otherwise he may demand inappropriately strict diabetic control, or too little control, depending on his unconscious needs to deny his own wound. The other author, a hemophiliac, has had difficulty mastering the biochemical mechanisms of blood coagulation. If wounds are left unconscious or poorly integrated into conscious awareness (Arrow 7), the quality of patient care (Arrow 2) may be adversely affected.

The helper's inner wound projections (Arrow 8) may occur more frequently in briefer and less introspective therapies conducted by healers of all professions. Within the psychologically oriented healing disciplines, however, projections seem less acceptable since greater self-understanding is expected. As suggested by the above case examples, strong emotions can be the stimulus for self reflection and uncovering of wounds. If the helper can remain open to and learn from the strong feelings created by the patient's wounds, greater awareness and integration of his own wounds may be realized.

Patient wounds are occasionally identified in their helpers (Arrow 9), whether actually present or not. For example, a male member of a small therapy group expressed concern over how the facilitator must be troubled by his crooked teeth. It was later shared by the group member that he was frequently worried about his physical appearance to the extent that meeting new people created great anxiety.

The conscious and direct support by the helper in regard to the patient's inner healer is a positive interaction facilitating the integration and increased awareness of the inner healer of the patient (Arrow 10). For example, a family having a recurrent problem may be reminded of past effective problem solving approaches used to remedy the problem and encouraged to focus on their healing family resources.

In another example, a woman patient with agorophobia and secondary alcoholism was being successfully treated for agorophobia although her life-threatening alcohol abuse continued. In a direct and caring manner, the therapist refused to continue treatment for the agorophobia unless the patient responsibly used her inner healing forces to discontinue drinking.

The mystery of healing interactions deepens when the interactions of the patient-healer and wounded-helper poles are considered (Arrows 11 and 12). The helper takes on the wounds of the patient (Arrow 1) and begins experiencing his own wounded polarity (Arrow 7), increasing an awareness of his own vulnerability. The helper's wounded pole activates and helps actualize the patient's healer pole, a step necessary for true healing (Arrow 12). Both patient and healer experience themselves more fully through greater awareness of their human potential to be both wounded and healed. This occurs both intrapersonally and interpersonally, ending in a greater sense of balance and wholeness for both individuals as both polarities are consciously experienced.

Unconscious interactions between patient and helper (Arrows 11 and 12) are also potentially harmful. As suggested by Langs (1985), patients may be more aware of the healer's wounds (Arrow 9) than the healer himself (Arrow 6). This awareness is rapidly repressed and the patient unknowingly becomes the healer (Arrow 11) in a role reversal which inappropriately benefits the professional healer and blocks progress for the patient. Langs conducted in-depth interviews with patients who had been in psychotherapy and discovered that many are unconsciously abused or manipulated to meet the needs of the professional healer. In such situations, neither patient nor professional are healed, even though the latter's needs may be briefly met.

However, when the patient experiences true healing, it often serves to heal the wounded pole of the professional healer (Arrow 11). In this case, there is mutual healing for both. This interaction will be addressed later in relation to professional burnout.

heal means whole

IMPLICATIONS FOR THE HEALING PROCESS

Wholeness

In considering the healing process, it is useful to consider the origins of the word heal, which derives from the Anglosaxon word hal, meaning whole. To heal, haelen, is to make whole (Webster's New Twentieth Century Dictionary, Second Edition, 1979). In general, factors facilitating healing also facilitate a sense of wholeness through the recognition and acceptance of all of one's parts and polarities. Gestalt therapy makes such integration a specific goal of therapy (Perls, Hefferline, & Goodman, 1951). Thus, healing and wholeness should be considered together.

Due to the constant distractions and demands of existence, a sense of wholeness in life is necessarily short-lived and elusive, even though one may expend much time and energy seeking it. A feeling or sense of wholeness often occurs with discovery or insight of hidden parts of oneself, e.g., finding an opposite pole leading to a greater sense of understanding and balance; the feeling of unity with another in sexual intercourse; the very transient sense of absurdity in a joke; the feeling of completeness when one experiences the dignity of a dying individual; and the sense of joy found in birth or a religious experience.

The authors believe that effective psychotherapy should contribute to healing and a greater sense of wholeness. Yalom (1980) has examined altruistic common denominators of effective psychotherapy as reflected in outcome research. He states that the effective therapist genuinely interacts with the patient, conveys warmth and empathy in a nonpossessive fashion, and grasps the meaning of the patient's life and experience. These qualities create an environment of such safety and acceptance that the patient can reveal those parts of himself which are usually hidden. Through therapy the patient learns to interact with all of his parts and becomes able to experience wholeness more frequently.

Conscious Inner Attention

Although these altruistic qualities are laudable and must be present to facilitate healing, the therapist must also learn to consciously attend to his inner self, if he is to truly attend to the inner self of his patient. Needleman (1985, pg. 84) believes this ability to be the secret of Freud's insight and creativity. He writes: "Freud had unconsciously discovered within himself the existence of a level and quality of human attention hitherto unsuspected and unrecognized by modern science, and found that this force of attention had not only served to balance Freud's own intellectual and emotional functions, thereby enabling him to be compassionate and insightful in the presence of his patients, but also that this force of attention itself 'radiated' to his patients a really effective healing influence, both in the sense of tangible healing energy and in the sense of calling forth in them the arising of their own self-mobilizing power of inner attention." As with Freud, it is through conscious inner attention, that the therapist most effectively heals his patients.

Conscious inner attention may be learned in psychotherapy or analysis during which unconscious elements emerge for examination. The practice of examining one's hidden self in the presence of another, soon becomes integrated and a part of the conscious inner attention useful to the effective healer. In Figure 1, all of the arrows arising from the healer's unconscious represent hidden conflicts which potentially clash with the patient's needs. The effective healer is aware of these conflicts in a way that promotes patient healing rather than detracting from it.

Vulnerability

We believe that conscious inner attention to one's wounds and conflicts leads to a sense of vulnerability. This, in turn, makes possible the unconscious connection between the healer's wound and the patient's healer (Arrows 11 and 12). As stated by Knight (1985), "the true healer cannot stand outside of the healing experience as a disinterested observer, but must be ready to have his or her own wounds activated and reactivated, but contained within and not projected." Through an encounter with the vulnerable healer, the patient finds more than temporary relief or alleviation of symptoms. Rather, the patient is able to go beyond his fears and resistances and discover the full meaning of his illness through a genuine understanding of the self. Weizsacker, as quoted by Jaspers (1964), states, "Only when the doctor has been deeply touched by the illness, infected by it, excited, frightened, shaken, only when it has been transferred to him, continues in him and is referred to himself by his own consciousness, only then and to that extent can he deal with it successfully." The genuine wounded-healer accepts his own wound along with that of the patient and finds therein an illumination which enables him to transcend the experience, while remaining forever both patient and healer.

Conscious attention to one's vulnerability may be augmented by the presence of a serious physical illness, particularly one which is chronic and unrelenting in nature. The literally wounded helper with such an illness is forced to attend to his own vulnerability and is likely to more humbly interact with his patients. The literally wounded helper is also likely to show greater empathy and understanding with the patient, since they share in common their woundedness.

Of greater significance, however, is the possibility that a literal wound in the helper may contribute, to the helper's own wholeness. After being afflicted by severe rheumatoid arthritis, Kreinheder (1980, pg. 15-17) wrote: "When you become ill, it is as if you have been chosen or elected, not as one to be limited and crippled, but as one to be healed. The disease always carries its own cure and also the cure for your whole personality. If you take it as your own and you stay with this new experience, with the pain and the fear and all the accompanying images, you will be healed to a wholeness far beyond your previous so-called health." In regard to the healing role, Kreinheder continues: "If you are going to be a healer, then you have to get into a relationship. There is a person before you, and you and that other person are there to relate. That means touching each other, touching the places in each other that are close and tender where the sensitivity is, where the wounds are, and where the turmoil is. That's intimacy. When you get this close, there is love. And when love comes, the healing comes. The therapist is an expert in the art of achieving intimacy. When you touch each other intimately and with good will, then there is healing."

However, Rippere and Williams (1985) discuss the tendency for many professional healers to wear a "protective mask" to keep patients at a distance. They claim patients respond positively to the "elusive quality of empathy" when healers remove their professional armour and reveal their vulnerability. The crucial factor of vulnerability, known for millennia, is frequently overlooked in the glitter of contemporary helper technology.

The contributions of Martin Buber (1958) in regard to facilitation of healing cannot be overstated. He characterizes the common form of human interaction as "I-It," where subject deals with object. This simple "I-It" relationship is unfortunately all too typical of many healer-patient interactions (Arrow 1 and 2). Buber decries this relationship as superficial and basically meaningless. In contrast, he describes the "I-Thou" relationship, in which each person is both subject and object and is able to recognize the totality of the other in this common experience. He believes that the greatest thing one human being can do for another is to confirm the deepest thing within him. Sometimes the deepest thing within healers are their wounds.

When a healer relates openly and totally with his patients, he models the I-Thou relationship which contributes to patient as well as healer wholeness. Also, when the healer pays attention to his own inner self, he can receive and follow clues provided by strong emotions, find the source of his personal wounds and experience his own vulnerability. If it is appropriate, the healer may, at times, share this information with patients. However, whether the process is shared or not, the humility and insight gained through such awareness is very important.

RELATED CONSIDERATIONS

Interest in the Healing Professions

In considering the motivation for entering the healing professions, one wonders if a sense of woundedness is not a major factor. Jung (1946) states, "the healer knows, or at least he should know that he did not choose his career by chance." Adler (1956) also claims, "To be wounded means also to have the healing power activated in us, or might we possibly say that without being wounded, one would never meet just this healing power, might we even go as far as to say that the very purpose of the wound is to make us aware of the healing power in us." Striking confirmation of these statements exist in the past history of substance abuse counselors, a large percentage of whom have been addicted. Their effectiveness in dealing with addicts may relate to the awareness of their own wounds.

Professional Burnout

As the healer consciously attends to his own vulnerability and deals with the pain of his patients, he becomes a receiver (Figure 1, Arrow 11). In other words, the healing encounter generates a flow of energy between patient and doctor, and this may be a sustaining source for true healers. Healers who cannot avail themselves of this profound source are more likely to experience loss of professional energy and effectiveness. If this is prolonged, it can result in burnout. Denial and repression of one's brokenness and vulnerability by itself may rob a healer of psychic energy and contribute to burnout. The act of affirming common human brokenness and vulnerability can bring life-giving energy and healing to both healer and patient.

It is hypothesized that burnout will probably be greater in professionals using more problem-oriented or technique oriented approaches, such as cognitive-behavioral approaches used by many psychologists, and medication-oriented or somatic treatments prescribed by psychiatrists. With these approaches, an "I-It" interaction is more likely to exist where the professional does not always attend or admit to his vulnerability. It is also hypothesized that healers using such approaches may over time discover a need to move toward other treatment modalities which allow the wounded aspects of themselves to be discovered and integrated.

Creativity

In discussing wholeness above, it was clearly implied that wholeness is closely associated with creativity. Indeed, moments of great psychic energy and joy appear to arise from acts of other or self-discovery and integration which provide a feeling of transcendence over the mundane finitude of our daily lives. These are the moments when polarities are reconciled and united and when wounds are healed. Such experiences of deep communion and understanding with ourselves or with others constitute a wellspring of truly creative insight and energy. We believe that the use of the self in therapy can result in such experiences of growth and creativity.

As in the ancient mythological figures who accomplished miracles despite their suffering, the wounded-healer remains creative and strong. His creativity is constantly renewed despite, or perhaps because of, his vulnerability. Nouwen (1972) may have had this in mind when he pointed out that "the creative man is always close to the abyss of sickness." In addition to facilitating healing, pain and suffering may be an effective stimulus for the creative process.

SUMMARY

In this communication, we have attempted to unravel the timeless mystery of healing. We have seen how wounded patients deny their inner healers as they search for and are treated by professional healers. We have also considered how role-bound professional healers deny and repress their own wounds while attempting to heal. Factors facilitating healing have been examined including the importance of conscious inner attention to and acceptance of one's own vulnerability.

From all these considerations, it appears that the therapist's acceptance of his own wounds through conscious awareness of his vulnerability contributes to a sense of wholeness, which in turn enables the patient to do the same and, thus, empowers his own healer.

NOTES

1. In preparing this paper, the authors frequently chose to name the acting individuals healer and patient. Despite the medical association of these words, this paradigm is useful for anyone involved in the helping professions, including counselors, social workers, family therapists, and psychologists. The word "patient" was used rather than "client," since most patients are more obviously wounded and this is not necessarily the case with clients. A heavy emphasis on the overt interaction between the patient and helper (Figure 1, Arrows 1 and 2) without awareness or consideration of helper woundedness may contribute to an inferior, dependent, or dehumanizing position for the patient. Some helping professionals have used the word "client" to remedy this situation. With the wounded-healer concept presented here, both helper and patient must humbly and mutually enter into the interaction for successful healing.

2. The authors purposely hyphenated the words wounded-healer even though literature references frequently do not. If left unhyphenated, the word wounded is subordinate and the wounded-healer polarity becomes less balanced. The unhyphenated approach may also contribute to the erroneous conclusion that we are discussing the "impaired physician."

REFERENCES

Adler, G. (1956). Notes regarding the dynamics of the self. In the *Collected Works*, 16, 111-125 (Bollingen, 1954). Princeton: Princeton University Press.

Buber, M. (1970). I and thou. New York: Scribners.

Fink, D. L. (1979). Holistic health: The evolution of Western medicine. In: *A humanistic perspective on holistic health values*. Grand Junction, CO: Western Colorado Health Systems Agency.

Graves, R. (1955). The Greek myths: Volume 1. New York: Penguin.

Groesbeck, C. J. (1975). The archetypal image of the wounded healer. *Journal of Analytical Psychology*, 20, 122-145.

Guggenbuhl-Craig, A. (1971). Power in the helping professions. Dallas: Spring.

Harner, M. (1980). The way of the shaman: A guide to power and healing. San Francisco: Harper and Row.

Jaspers, J. (1964). The nature of psychotherapy: A critical appraisal. Chicago: University of Chicago.

Johnson, R. A. (1974). He—understanding masculine psychology. New York: Harper and Row.

Jung, C. G. (1946). Psychology of the transference. In the *Collected Works*, 16, 133-338 (Bollingen, 1954). Princeton: Princeton University Press.

Jung, C. G. (1951). Fundamental questions of psychotherapy. In the *Collected Works*, 16, 111-125 (Bollingen, 1954). Princeton: Princeton University Press.

Kerenyi, C. (1959). Asklepios, archetypal image of the physician's existence. Translated by Ralph Manheim (Bollingen Series LXV). Princeton: Princeton University Press.

Knight, J. A. (1985). Religio-psychological dimensions of wounded healers. Presented at the annual meeting of the American Psychiatric Association, Dallas, Texas, May 20.

Kreinheder, A. (1980). The healing power of illness. *Psychological Perspectives*, Spring 11(1), 9-18.

Langs, R. (1985). Madness and cure. New York: New Concept Press.

Meyerhoff, B. G. (1976). Balancing between worlds: The shaman's calling. *Parabola*, 1, 6-13.

Needlcham, J. (1985). The way of the physician. New York: Harper and Row.

Nouwen, H. J. M. (1972). The wounded healer—ministry in contemporary society. Garden City, NY: Image.

Plato (1951). The symposium. Translated by W. Hamilton. New York: Penguin.

Perls, F., Hefferline, R.F., & Goodman, P. (1951). Gestalt therapy: Excitement and growth in the human personality. New York: Dell.

Rippere, V. & Williams, R. (1985). Wounded healers. Chichester: John Wiley and Sons.

Webster's New Twentieth Century Unabridged Dictionary, Second Edition (1979). New York: Simon and Shuster.

Yalom, I. D. (1980). Existential psychotherapy. New York: Basic Books.

Epilogue

Psychotherapy must be understood within the larger framework of the society within which it exists. Changes that we believe are taking place in psychotherapy are also taking place at the cutting edge of other fields as the ideas of scientists regarding the limitations of a purely objective and technological approach to life trickle into the main stream of society. These ideas have not usually come from behavioral scientists, psychiatrists or theologians, but from prominent scientists in the most basic disciplines, such as physics, mathematics, chemistry, molecular genetics. They became aware that pure objectivity is an illusion, that objects are changed by the very process of observation (Heisenberg's uncertainty principle, 1927), and that not everything which exists is observable (Lynch, 1977). Paradoxically, these discoveries were made at a time when belief in science and technology was a dominant societal trend. However, as the limitations of a technological approach become more evident, the pendulum is beginning to swing in the opposite direction in areas such as medicine (Cousins, 1983), and business (Naisbitt, 1982).

The papers in this collection on the "Use of Self," have covered issues ranging from broad philosophical discussions of the nature of the self to the personal thoughts and feelings of psychotherapists as they reflect upon their experience. The viewpoints expressed reflect some doubts about the universal applicability of the scientific method to all human problems. It appears clear that the importance of therapeutic techniques cannot overshadow the fact that the self of the therapist is the funnel through which theories and techniques become manifest. This holds true regardless of the therapeutic modality. Indeed, there would not be any group or family therapy without individual human beings. In most instances, individuals in therapy are in pain and feel lonely. Yet pain and loneliness are not reached by techniques alone. As Yalom points out along with many others, "it is the relationship that heals. Every therapist observes over and over in clinical work that the encounter itself is healing for the patient in a way that transcends the therapist's theoretical orientation" (1980, p. 401). The self is always present in therapy, even when it is denied.

THE NEED FOR AN EDUCATED SELF

What are the implications of a belief that the self of the therapist is central to the therapeutic process? One important conclusion is that it needs to be a major focus of attention from both a clinical and training standpoint. Mauksch, in an unpublished paper (1986), suggests that if the Self is considered to be an essential resource, it deserves to be looked upon from the perspective of a technological model of resources management. The use of this precious resource, then, warrants and deserves the application of skills, care and maintenance. When one contemplates the expenditure of efforts, thought and time which go into learning how to use a computer, it is ludicrous to think of the scant attention paid to the use of this most complex of instruments, the Self.

A major consideration is the protection of the client. Since the Self has a potential for negative as well as positive impact, our first guide should be Hippocrates' dictum "First of all do no harm." In his recent book, *Madness and Cure*, Robert Langs (1986) reminds us of the dangers of the loosely-structured treatment framework which guides a great deal of psychotherapy being practiced today. The clinical data which he reports illustrates the degree to which the therapeutic relationship can be grossly misused in the service of the therapist's own uncontained needs. Even though one may not agree with many of Langs' psychoanalytic interpretations, his caution to the therapist regarding the possible negative impact of the self should encourage us to re-envision the therapeutic task, and to question the possibility of harming the client or patient through misuse of the self.

As Aponte and Winter point out in their paper, the family therapist is even less protected than the analyst from imposing his own personal values and life issues on the patient, especially if the patient's difficulties resonate with those of the therapist. The role of the family therapist demands enormous personal self-knowledge and discipline from the practitioner.

IMPLICATIONS FOR TRAINING

We would like to see training programs reflect the fact that the self of the therapist is the means through which theories and techniques become manifest: "The growth of the self is fostered through education, guidance, encouragement, and above all, through respectful recognition and support" (Mauksch 1986). When training programs ignore this, the implied message to the trainee is that such ability is either unimportant, innate or involves skills so easy or difficult as to be ignored by the training program. Some programs may operate on the assumption that they teach about the use of self when in actuality they are focusing on skills and techniques. Learning about the self is extremely delicate, as such skills and sensitivities are difficult to define in conventional terms. It also puts additional pressures on the faculty, since it exposes them to the threat of looking within and having to deal with their own vulnerabilities. Another difficulty with emphasizing the use of self in training programs stems from the fact that the self is only able to flourish in a non-judgemental framework—parallel to what goes on in therapy—and requires from the trainer the willingness to let go of control and to flow with the discovery process.

The development of the self of the therapist must be a continuous and ongoing process. Although the foregoing statement seems obvious, it is easy to fall into a routine of daily life and work which denies the time and energy needed for the nurture of the self. The consequences of such neglect are unfortunate. Indeed, when the therapist ignores the development of the internal processes which enable him to recognize and deal with destructive elements, he is unable to model for his clients the integration of positive growth processes which are at the heart of the therapeutic process (Luthman & Kirschenbaum, 1974). An alive and vibrant self is a source of energy and creativity which is of benefit to the therapeutic encounter as well as to the well-being of the therapist. When the therapist maintains such a direct person-to-person contact with his patients, his energies are renewed and the danger of burn-out is lessened.

This presentation of viewpoints on the use of self in therapy makes no claim for originality or innovation. It is our belief that effective therapy throughout history has embodied this concept and that effective therapists have exhibited this quality in their most healing and helpful moments. Rather, our plea is for a more conscious recognition and awareness of its importance in the therapeutic process and for a greater emphasis on the development and nurture of this remarkable therapeutic tool.

NOTE

1. We purposely chose the expression "need for an educated self" rather than "need for training the self" because the word training could imply a mechanistic or technical approach.

REFERENCES

Cousins, N. (1983). *The Healing Heart*. New York: W.W. Norton.
Langs, R. (1985). *Madness and Cure*. New Concept Press.
Luthman, S.G., & Kirschenbaum, M. (1974). *The Dynamic Family*. Palo Alto: Science and Behavior Books.
Lynch J.J. (1977). *The Broken Heart*. Basic Books, Inc.
Mauksch, H.O. (1986). *Use of Self: Towards a Technology of Helping*. Unpublished manuscript.
Naisbitt, J. (1982). *Megatrends*. New York: Warner Books.
Yalom I.D. (1980). *Existential Psychotherapy*. New York: Basic Books, Inc.